DELIBERATE PRACTICE IN
SCHEMA
THERAPY

Essentials of Deliberate Practice Series

Tony Rousmaniere and Alexandre Vaz, Series Editors

ESSENTIALS OF DELIBERATE PRACTICE SERIES
TONY ROUSMANIERE AND ALEXANDRE VAZ, SERIES EDITORS

DELIBERATE PRACTICE IN
SCHEMA THERAPY

WENDY T. BEHARY
JOAN M. FARRELL
ALEXANDRE VAZ
TONY ROUSMANIERE

AMERICAN PSYCHOLOGICAL ASSOCIATION

Published by
American Psychological Association
750 First Street, NE
Washington, DC 20002
https://www.apa.org

Order Department
https://www.apa.org/pubs/books
order@apa.org

In the U.K., Europe, Africa, and the Middle East, copies may be ordered from Eurospan
https://www.eurospanbookstore.com/apa
info@eurospangroup.com

Typeset in Cera Pro by Circle Graphics, Inc., Reisterstown, MD

Printer: Gasch Printing, Odenton, MD
Cover Designer: Mark Karis

Library of Congress Cataloging-in-Publication Data

Names: Behary, Wendy T., author. | Farrell, Joan M., author. | Vaz, Alexandre, author. |
   Rousmaniere, Tony, author. | American Psychological Association.
Title: Deliberate practice in schema therapy / Wendy T. Behary, Joan M. Farrell,
   Alexandre Vaz, and Tony Rousmaniere.
Description: Washington, DC : American Psychological Association, 2023. |
   Series: Essentials of deliberate practice series | Includes
   bibliographical references and index.
Identifiers: LCCN 2022027881 (print) | LCCN 2022027882 (ebook) |
   ISBN 9781433836022 (paperback) | ISBN 9781433836039 (ebook)
Subjects: LCSH: Schemas (Psychology) | Schema-focused cognitive therapy.
Classification: LCC BF313 .B44 2023 (print) | LCC BF313 (ebook) |
   DDC 153--dc23/eng/20220824
LC record available at https://lccn.loc.gov/2022027881
LC ebook record available at https://lccn.loc.gov/2022027882

https://doi.org/10.1037/0000326-000

Printed in the United States of America

10 9 8 7 6 5 4 3 2 1

Contents

Series Preface

Tony Rousmaniere and Alexandre Vaz

We are pleased to introduce the Essentials of Deliberate Practice series of training books. We are developing this book series to address a specific need that we see in many psychology training programs. The issue can be illustrated by the training experiences of Mary, a hypothetical second-year graduate school trainee. Mary has learned a lot about mental health theory, research, and psychotherapy techniques. Mary is a dedicated student; she has read dozens of textbooks, has written excellent papers about psychotherapy, and receives near-perfect scores on her course exams. However, when Mary sits with her clients at her practicum site, she often has trouble performing the therapy skills that she can write and talk about so clearly. Furthermore, Mary has noticed herself getting anxious when her clients express strong reactions, such as getting very emotional, hopeless, or skeptical about therapy. Sometimes this anxiety is strong enough to make Mary freeze at key moments, limiting her ability to help those clients.

During her weekly individual and group supervision, Mary's supervisor gives her advice informed by empirically supported therapies and common factor methods. The supervisor often supplements that advice by leading Mary through role-plays, recommending additional reading, or providing examples from her own work with clients. Mary, a dedicated supervisee who shares tapes of her sessions with her supervisor, is open about her challenges, carefully writes down her supervisor's advice, and reads the suggested readings. However, when Mary sits back down with her clients, she often finds that her new knowledge seems to have flown out of her head, and she is unable to enact her supervisor's advice. Mary finds this problem to be particularly acute with the clients who are emotionally evocative.

Mary's supervisor, who has received formal training in supervision, uses supervisory best practices, including the use of video to review supervisees' work. She would rate Mary's overall competence level as consistent with expectations for a trainee at Mary's developmental level. But even though Mary's overall progress is positive, she experiences some recurring problems in her work. This is true even though the supervisor is confident that she and Mary have identified the changes that Mary should make in her work.

The problem with which Mary and her supervisor are wrestling—the disconnect between her knowledge about psychotherapy and her ability to reliably perform psychotherapy—is the focus of this book series. We started this series because most therapists experience this disconnect, to one degree or another, whether they are beginning trainees or highly experienced clinicians. In truth, we are all Mary.

To address this problem, we are focusing this series on the use of deliberate practice, a method of training specifically designed for improving reliable performance of complex skills in challenging work environments (Rousmaniere, 2016, 2019; Rousmaniere et al., 2017). Deliberate practice entails experiential, repeated training with a particular skill until it becomes automatic. In the context of psychotherapy, this involves two trainees role-playing as a client and a therapist, switching roles every so often, under the guidance of a supervisor. The trainee playing the therapist reacts to client statements, ranging in difficulty from beginner to intermediate to advanced, with improvised responses that reflect fundamental therapeutic skills.

To create these books, we approached leading trainers and researchers of major therapy models with these simple instructions: Identify 10 to 12 essential skills for your therapy model where trainees often experience a disconnect between cognitive knowledge and performance ability—in other words, skills that trainees could write a good paper about but often have challenges performing, especially with challenging clients. We then collaborated with the authors to create deliberate practice exercises specifically designed to improve reliable performance of these skills and overall responsive treatment (Hatcher, 2015; Stiles et al., 1998; Stiles & Horvath, 2017). Finally, we rigorously tested these exercises with trainees and trainers at multiple sites around the world and refined them based on extensive feedback.

Each book in this series focuses on a specific therapy model, but readers will notice that most exercises in these books touch on common factor variables and facilitative interpersonal skills that researchers have identified as having the most impact on client outcome, such as empathy, verbal fluency, emotional expression, persuasiveness, and problem focus (e.g., Anderson et al., 2009; Norcross et al., 2019). Thus, the exercises in every book should help with a broad range of clients. Despite the specific theoretical model(s) from which therapists work, most therapists place a strong emphasis on pantheoretical elements of the therapeutic relationship, many of which have robust empirical support as correlates or mechanisms of client improvement (e.g., Norcross et al., 2019). We also recognize that therapy models have already-established training programs with rich histories, so we present deliberate practice not as a replacement but as an adaptable, transtheoretical training method that can be integrated into these existing programs to improve skill retention and help ensure basic competency.

About This Book

This book is focused on schema therapy, an approach that evolved from the work of Jeffrey Young and others with a focus on more effectively treating clients with personality disorders and those with chronic symptom profiles who failed to respond to or relapsed after traditional cognitive behavioral therapy (Arntz, 1994; Behary, 2008, 2021; Farrell et al., 2014; Farrell & Shaw, 1994, 2012; Young, 1990; Young et al., 2003). Young's theoretical–conceptual framework originally focused on individual therapy (Young, 1990; Young et al., 2003) and was later adapted to also work with couples, groups, and children and adolescents. Schema therapy is a comprehensive, clear, and robust theoretical model—one that strategically selects and integrates strategies from other psychotherapy schools of thought, such as cognitive behavioral, gestalt, and emotion-focused therapies; eye movement desensitization and reprocessing; mindfulness; interpersonal neurobiology; and somatosensory interventions.

Our goal with this book is for deliberate practice to be an additional piece designed to enhance schema therapy training. Ideally, deliberate practice can help trainees and therapists integrate essential schema therapy skills into their repertoire, allowing access to them in an automatic fashion in response to the client context. The skills set forth in this book are the basic skills; they are not intended to be comprehensive. Deliberate practice is not intended to be the only training format through which schema therapy competency is acquired. It is best viewed as an important new complement to other training and supervision methods.

Thank you for including us in your journey toward psychotherapy expertise. Now let's get to practice!

Acknowledgments

We would like to acknowledge Rodney Goodyear for his significant contribution to starting and organizing this book series. We are grateful to Susan Reynolds, David Becker, Emily Ekle, and Joe Albrecht at American Psychological Association (APA) Books and Elizabeth Budd for providing expert guidance and insightful editing that has significantly improved the quality and accessibility of this book. We would also like to acknowledge the International Deliberate Practice Society and its members for their many contributions and support for our work. Finally, we are grateful for the invaluable editorial notes and feedback from Inês Amaro, Amy DeSmidt, and Jamie Manser.

We are grateful to Jeff Young and Ida Shaw for their unwavering support and contributions. We are also grateful to our colleagues and trainees from the International Society of Schema Therapy for your inspiration and enthusiasm. Finally, we want to acknowledge our patients for the privilege of knowing them and witnessing their courage.

The exercises in this book underwent extensive testing at training programs around the world. For all the pilot site leaders and trainees who volunteered to "test run" this work and provided critically important feedback throughout the method refinement and writing process, we cannot thank you enough. In particular, we are deeply grateful to the following supervisors and trainees who tested exercises and provided invaluable feedback:

- Diana Bandeira, MR Terapias, Lisboa, Portugal
- Myriam Bechtoldt, private practice, Frankfurt, Germany
- Marsha Blank, private practice, Brooklyn, NY, United States
- Shana Dastur, private practice, Caldwell, NJ, United States
- Joana David, Clínica ISPA, Lisboa, Portugal
- Aleksandra Defranc, University of Warsaw, Warsaw, Poland
- Tara Cutland Green, private practice, East Riding of Yorkshire, England, United Kingdom
- Max Groth, private practice, New York, NY, United States
- Johanna Knorr, private practice, Kassel, Germany
- Anna-Maija Kokko, Center for Cognitive Psychotherapy Luote Ltd, Mikkeli, Finland
- Nicolette Kulp, SAGA Community Center, Ambler, PA, United States
- Zhi Li, private practice, Rotterdam, The Netherlands
- Christopher Lin and Danni Hang, Ferkauf Graduate School of Psychology, Bronx, NY, United States

- Offer Maurer, private practice, Cascais, Portugal
- Pam Pilkington, private practice, Melbourne, Australia
- Nicholas Scheidt, private practice, Miami Beach, FL, United States
- Robin Spiro, private practice, Livingston, NJ, United States
- Marieke ten Napel-Schutz, Radboud University, Rozendaal, The Netherlands
- Mingxin Wei, private practice, Baltimore, MD, United States
- Yuanchen Zhu, private practice, Shanghai, China

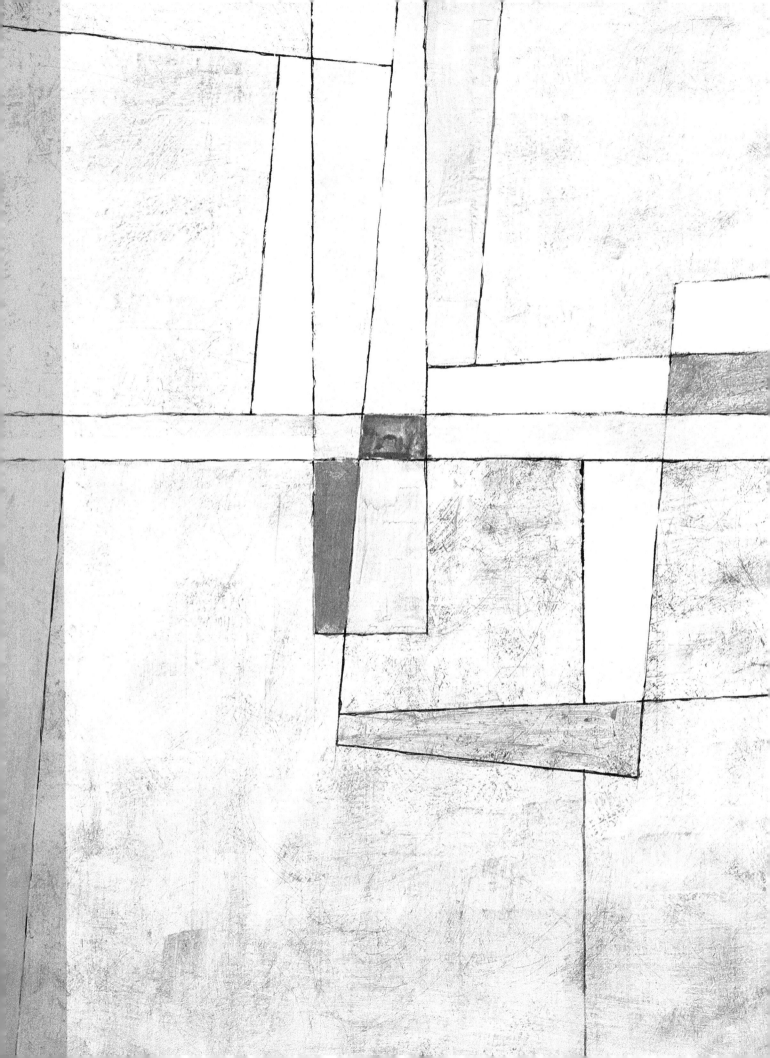

Overview and Instructions

In Part I, we provide an overview of deliberate practice, including how it can be integrated into clinical training programs for schema therapy (ST), and instructions for performing the deliberate practice exercises in Part II. **We encourage both trainers and trainees to read both Chapters 1 and 2 before performing the deliberate practice exercises for the first time.**

Chapter 1 provides a foundation for the rest of the book by introducing important concepts related to deliberate practice and its role in psychotherapy training more broadly and ST training more specifically. We also review the 12 skills included in the deliberate practice exercises.

Chapter 2 lays out the basic, most essential instructions for performing the ST deliberate practice exercises in Part II. They are designed to be quick and simple and provide you with just enough information to get started without being overwhelmed by too much information. Chapter 3 in Part III provides more in-depth guidance, which we encourage you to read once you are comfortable with the basic instructions in Chapter 2.

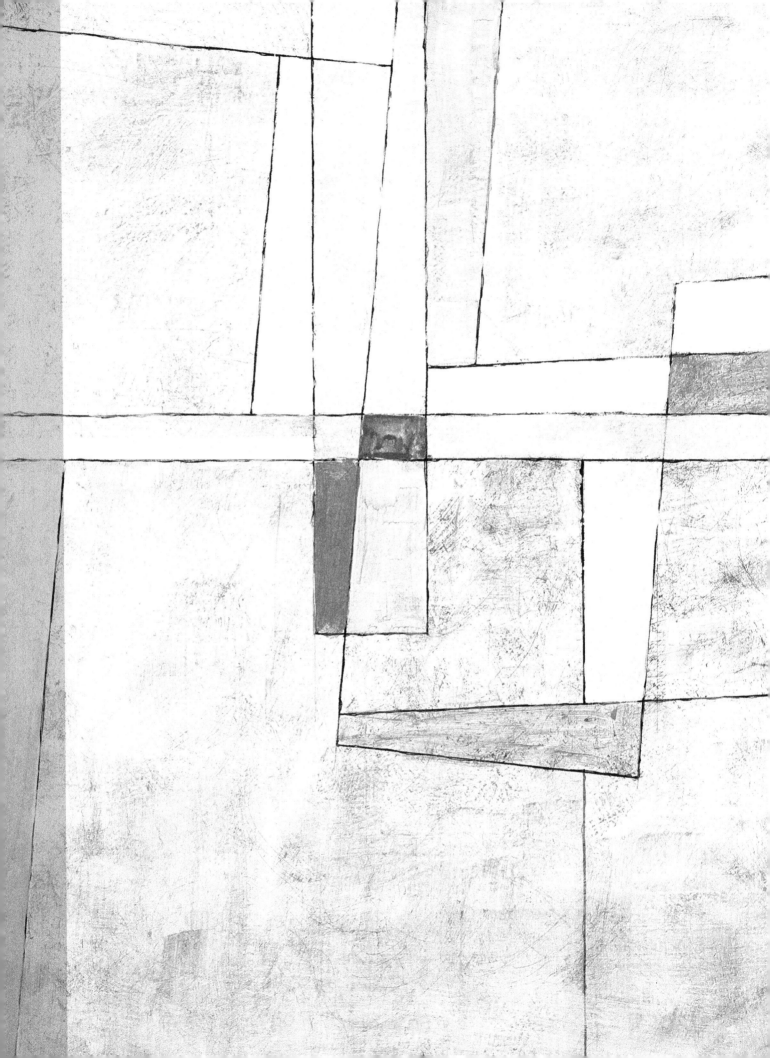

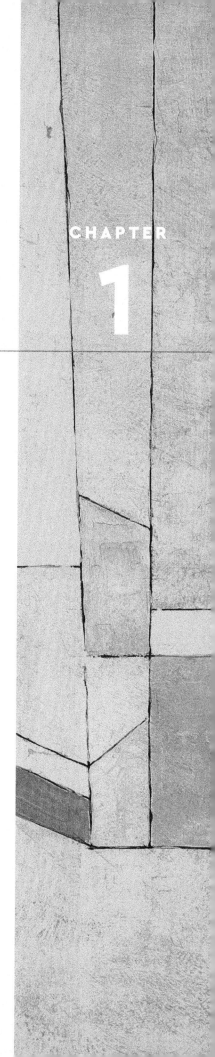

Introduction and Overview of Deliberate Practice and Schema Therapy

My (W. T. B.) personal exposure to schema therapy (ST) began with the privilege of learning and working alongside Jeff Young, and other colleagues, in the early development of the model. There was discussion, experimentation, and procedural attention paid to theory, conceptualization, treatment formulation, and application. Deliberate practice, with its targeted microskills learning, would have added value to training competent ST practitioners. In this book, we want to fill this common gap in therapists' procedural training. The focused attention that deliberate practice pays to breaking down complex interventions into small parts offers clinicians the opportunity to practice skills carefully in the context of specific problems. Repetitive practice, so often missing in psychotherapy training, is a prerequisite to developing professional expertise and flexibility in many other fields. In learning tennis, focused attention must go into experiencing each part of the execution: posture, grip, footing, timing, eye contact, and follow-through. Then it's practice, practice, practice. Eventually, the relationship with the racquet in hand and your placement on the court is formed. Much in the same way, we believe that mindfulness and deliberate skills practice are necessary elements to develop competent schema therapists.

Overview of the Deliberate Practice Exercises

The main focus of the book is a series of 14 exercises that have been thoroughly tested by an international community of ST trainers and trainees. Each of the first 12 exercises represents an essential ST skill. The last two exercises are more comprehensive, consisting of an annotated ST transcript and improvised mock therapy sessions that teach practitioners how to integrate all these skills into more expansive clinical scenarios. Table 1.1 presents the 12 skills that are covered in these exercises.

Throughout all the exercises, trainees work in pairs under the guidance of a supervisor and role-play as a client and a therapist, switching back and forth between the two roles. Each of the 12 skill-focused exercises consists of multiple client statements grouped by

https://doi.org/10.1037/0000326-001

TABLE 1.1. The 12 Schema Therapy Skills Presented in the Deliberate Practice Exercises

Beginner Skills	Intermediate Skills	Advanced Skills
1. Understanding and attunement 2. Supporting and strengthening the healthy adult mode 3. Schema education: beginning to understand current problems in schema therapy terms 4. Linking unmet needs, schema, and presenting problem	5. Education about maladaptive schema modes 6. Recognizing the mode shifts of the maladaptive coping modes 7. Identifying the presence of the demanding/ punitive inner critic mode 8. Identifying the presence of the angry and vulnerable child modes	9. Limited reparenting for the angry and vulnerable child modes 10. Limited reparenting for the demanding/ punitive inner critic mode 11. Limited reparenting for the maladaptive coping modes: empathic confrontation 12. Implementing behavioral pattern breaking through homework assignments

difficulty—beginner, intermediate, and advanced—that calls for a specific skill. For each skill, trainees are asked to read through and absorb the description of the skill, its criteria, and some examples of it. The trainee playing the client then reads the statements. The trainee playing the therapist then responds in a way that demonstrates the appropriate skill. Trainee therapists will have the option of practicing a response using the one supplied in the exercise or immediately improvising and supplying their own.

After each client statement and therapist response couplet is practiced several times, the trainees will stop to receive feedback from the supervisor. Guided by the supervisor, the trainees will be instructed to try statement–response couplets several times, working their way down the list. In consultation with the supervisor, trainees will go through the exercises, starting with the least challenging and moving through to more advanced levels. The triad (supervisor–client–therapist) will have the opportunity to discuss whether exercises present too much or too little challenge and adjust up or down depending on the assessment.

Trainees, in consultation with supervisors, can decide which skills they wish to work on and for how long. On the basis of our testing experience, we have found that, to receive maximum benefit, practice sessions should last about 1 to 1.25 hours. After this, trainees become saturated and need a break.

Ideally, ST learners will both gain confidence and achieve competence through practicing these exercises. *Competence* is defined here as the ability to perform an ST skill in a manner that is flexible and responsive to the client. Skills have been chosen that are considered essential to ST and that practitioners often find challenging to implement.

The skills identified in this book are not comprehensive in the sense of representing all one needs to learn to become a competent ST clinician. Some will present particular challenges for trainees.

The Goals of This Book

The primary goal of this book is to help trainees achieve competence in core ST skills. Therefore, the expression of that skill or competency may look somewhat different across clients or even within session with the same client.

The deliberate practice exercises are designed to accomplish the following:

1. Help schema therapists develop the ability to apply the skills in a range of clinical situations.

2. Move the skills into procedural memory (Squire, 2004) so that schema therapists can access them even when they are tired, stressed, overwhelmed, or discouraged.

3. Provide schema-therapists-in-training with an opportunity to exercise skills using a style and language that is congruent with who they are.

4. Provide the opportunity to use the ST skills in response to varying client statements and affect. This is designed to build confidence to adopt skills in a broad range of circumstances within different client contexts.

5. Provide schema therapists in training with many opportunities to fail and then correct their failed response based on feedback. This helps build confidence and persistence.

Finally, this book aims to help trainees discover their own personal learning style so they can continue their professional development long after their formal training is concluded.

Who Can Benefit From This Book?

This book is designed to be used in multiple contexts, including in graduate-level courses, supervision, postgraduate training, training for the International Society of Schema Therapy certification, and continuing education programs. It assumes the following:

1. The trainer is knowledgeable about and competent in ST.

2. The trainer can provide good demonstrations of how to use ST skills across a range of therapeutic situations, via role-play, or the trainer has access to examples of ST being demonstrated through psychotherapy video recordings.

3. The trainer can provide feedback to students regarding how to craft or improve their application of ST skills.

4. Trainees will have accompanying reading, such as books and articles, that explain the theory, research, and rationale of ST and each particular skill.

The exercises covered in this book were piloted at 19 training sites from across four continents (North America, Europe, Asia, and Oceania). This book is designed for trainers and trainees from different cultural backgrounds worldwide.

This book is also designed for those who are training at all career stages, from beginning trainees, including those who have never worked with real clients, to seasoned therapists. All exercises feature guidance for assessing and adjusting the difficulty to precisely target the needs of each individual learner. The term *trainee* in this book is used broadly, referring to anyone in the field of professional mental health who is endeavoring to acquire ST skills.

Deliberate Practice in Psychotherapy Training

How does one become an expert in their professional field? What is trainable, and what is simply beyond our reach, due to innate or uncontrollable factors? Questions such as these touch on our fascination with expert performers and their development. A mixture of awe, admiration, and even confusion surround people such as Mozart, Leonardo da Vinci, and more contemporary top performers such as basketball legend Michael Jordan and chess virtuoso Garry Kasparov. What accounts for their consistently superior professional results? Evidence suggests that the amount of time spent on a particular type of training is a key factor in developing expertise in virtually all domains (Ericsson & Pool, 2016). "Deliberate practice" is an evidence-based method that can improve performance in an effective and reliable manner.

The concept of deliberate practice has its origins in a classic study by K. Anders Ericsson and colleagues (1993), who found that the amount of time practicing a skill and the quality of the time spent doing so were key factors predicting mastery and acquisition. They identified five key activities in learning and mastering skills: (a) observing one's own work, (b) getting expert feedback, (c) setting small incremental learning goals just beyond the performer's ability, (d) engaging in repetitive behavioral rehearsal of specific skills, and (e) continuously assessing performance. Ericsson and his colleagues termed this process *deliberate practice*, a cyclical process that is illustrated in Figure 1.1.

Research has shown that lengthy engagement in deliberate practice is associated with expert performance across a variety of professional fields, such as medicine, sports, music, chess, computer programming, and mathematics (Ericsson et al., 2018). People may associate deliberate practice with the widely known "10,000-hour rule" popularized by Malcolm Gladwell in his 2008 book, *Outliers*, although the actual number of hours required for expertise varies by field and by individual (Ericsson & Pool, 2016). This, though, perpetuated two misunderstandings—first, that this is the number of deliberate practice hours that everyone needs to attain expertise, no matter the domain. In fact, there can be considerable variability in how many hours are required. The second misunderstanding is that engagement in 10,000 hours of work performance will lead one to become an expert in that domain. This misunderstanding holds considerable significance for the field of psychotherapy, where hours of work experience with clients

FIGURE 1.1. Cycle of Deliberate Practice

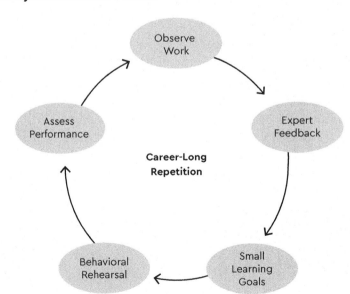

Note. From *Deliberate Practice in Emotion-Focused Therapy* (p. 7), by R. N. Goldman, A. Vaz, and T. Rousmaniere, 2021, American Psychological Association (https://doi.org/10.1037/0000227-000). Copyright 2021 by the American Psychological Association.

has traditionally been used as a measure of proficiency (Rousmaniere, 2016). Research suggests that the amount of experience alone does not predict therapist effectiveness (Goldberg, Babins-Wagner, et al., 2016; Goldberg, Rousmaniere, et al., 2016). It may be that the quality of deliberate practice is a key factor.

Psychotherapy scholars, recognizing the value of deliberate practice in other fields, have recently called for deliberate practice to be incorporated into training for mental health professionals (e.g., Bailey & Ogles, 2019; Hill et al., 2020; Rousmaniere et al., 2017; Taylor & Neimeyer, 2017; Tracey et al., 2015). There are, however, good reasons to question analogies made between psychotherapy and other professional fields, like sports or music, because by comparison psychotherapy is so complex and free form. Sports have clearly defined goals, and classical music follows a written score. In contrast, the goals of psychotherapy shift with the unique presentation of each client at each session. Therapists do not have the luxury of following a score.

Instead, good psychotherapy is more like improvisational jazz (Noa Kageyama, as cited in Rousmaniere, 2016). In jazz improvisations, a complex mixture of group collaboration, creativity, and interaction are coconstructed among band members. Like psychotherapy, no two jazz improvisations are identical. However, improvisations are not a random collection of notes. They are grounded in a comprehensive theoretical understanding and technical proficiency that is only developed through continuous deliberate practice. For example, prominent jazz instructor Jerry Coker (1990) lists 18 skill areas that students must master, each of which has multiple discrete skills, including tone quality, intervals, chord arpeggios, scales, patterns, and licks. In this sense, more creative and artful improvisations are actually a reflection of a previous commitment to repetitive skill practice and acquisition. As legendary jazz musician Miles Davis put it, "You have to play a long time to be able to play like yourself" (Cook, 2005).

The main idea that we would like to stress here is that we want deliberate practice to help schema therapists become themselves. The idea is to learn the skills so that you have them on hand when you want them. Practice the skills to make them your own. Incorporate those aspects that feel right for you. Ongoing and effortful deliberate practice should not be an impediment to flexibility and creativity. Ideally, it should enhance them. We recognize and celebrate that psychotherapy is an ever-shifting encounter and by no means want it to become or feel formulaic. Strong schema therapists mix an eloquent integration of previously acquired skills with properly attuned flexibility. The core ST responses provided are meant as templates or possibilities, rather than "answers." Please interpret and apply them as you see fit, in a way that makes sense to you. We encourage flexible and improvisational play!

Simulation-Based Mastery Learning

Deliberate practice uses simulation-based mastery learning (Ericsson, 2004; McGaghie et al., 2014). That is, the stimulus material for training consists of "contrived social situations that mimic problems, events, or conditions that arise in professional encounters" (McGaghie et al., 2014, p. 375). A key component of this approach is that the stimuli being used in training are sufficiently similar to the real-world experiences that they provoke similar reactions. This facilitates *state-dependent learning*, where professionals acquire skills in the same psychological environment where they will ultimately perform them (Fisher & Craik, 1977; Smith, 1979). For example, pilots train with flight simulators that present mechanical failures and dangerous weather conditions, and surgeons practice with surgical simulators that present medical complications. Training in simulations with challenging stimuli increases professionals' capacity to perform effectively under stress. For the psychotherapy training exercises in this book, the "simulators" are typical client statements that might actually be presented in the course of therapy sessions and call upon the use of the particular skill.

Declarative Versus Procedural Knowledge

Declarative knowledge is what a person can understand, write, or speak about. It often refers to factual information that can be consciously recalled through memory and often acquired relatively quickly. In contrast, procedural learning is implicit in memory, and "usually requires *repetition of an activity*, and associated learning is demonstrated through *improved task performance*" (Koziol & Budding, 2012, pp. 2694, emphasis added). *Procedural knowledge* is what a person can perform, especially under stress (Squire, 2004). There can be a wide difference between their declarative and procedural knowledge. For example, an "armchair quarterback" is a person who understands and talks about athletics well but would have trouble performing it at a professional level. Likewise, most dance, music, or theater critics have a very high ability to write about their subjects but would be flummoxed if asked to perform them.

The sweet spot for deliberate practice is the gap between declarative and procedural knowledge. In other words, effortful practice should target those skills that the trainee could write a good paper about but would have trouble actually performing with a real client. We start with declarative knowledge, learning skills theoretically and observing others perform them. Once learned, with the help of deliberate practice, we work toward the development of procedural learning, with the aim of therapists having "automatic" access to each of the skills that they can pull on when necessary.

Let us turn to the theoretical background on ST to help contextualize the skills of the book and how they fit into the greater training model.

Overview of Schema Therapy

ST, informed by and compatible with developmental psychology theory and research on attachment (summarized in Cassidy & Shaver, 1999) and interpersonal neurobiology (Siegel, 1999), is unique in its strategic integration of experiential, cognitive, and behavioral pattern-breaking interventions, as opposed to general eclectic approaches. The integrative approach of ST may account for the significant effect sizes found in individual and group treatment outcome studies (e.g., Farrell et al., 2009; Giesen-Bloo et al., 2006). These studies demonstrated symptom reduction, improved global functioning, and meaningful, sustainable, personality changes.

Core Concepts

ST proposes that difficulties in adult life may be linked with unmet core emotional needs in childhood. These basic needs are identified as follows:

- secure attachment/connection to others (includes affection, empathy, safety, stability, nurturance, and acceptance)
- support for autonomy, competence, and sense of identity
- freedom and assertiveness, to express valid needs, thoughts, opinions, and emotions spontaneity and play
- realistic limits and self-control

Early maladaptive schemas (EMSs)—the personality traits that include unchallenged and rigidly embedded maladaptive "truths" (beliefs about ourselves, the world, and our relationships with other people)—may form in response to these unmet needs, carrying intense emotion, rigid beliefs, and bodily sensations, as well as impulses to react, when triggered by conditions that resemble early life experiences, to shut down the unbearable pain associated with EMS activation.

Psychological disorders can be described and understood in terms of the operation of schemas and modes. The concept of modes offers the client and the clinician user-friendly language for identifying these self-defeating patterns of behavior. Aggression, hostility, manipulation, dominance, approval seeking, stimulation seeking, substance abuse, overcompliance, dependence, excessive self-reliance, compulsivity, inhibition, social isolation, and emotional avoidance, as well as internalized demanding, critical, and punishing modes, can all be understood in mode terms as self-defeating responses to schema activation or as internalized self-critical, self-demanding, or self-punishing messages. Clients suffering from severe personality disorders switch modes more frequently because of higher sensitivity to environmental, interpersonal, and intrapersonal triggers, causing sudden behavioral shifts and overly intense reactions. Modes can also stay rigidly entrenched as default ways of being, as in the case of many avoidant clients.

EMSs are thought to result from the interactions of unmet core childhood needs, innate temperament, and other early environmental experiences—nature and nurture. They become the implicitly driven ways of relating to the world under specific and familiar conditions—that is, a blueprint for life and a sense of how the world works. The 18 EMSs identified by Young, which are presented in Appendix C, are based on hypothesized basic needs of childhood (Young et al., 2003). In ST, the definition of EMS is broader than that of cognitive behavior therapy because it includes memories, bodily sensations, emotions, and cognitions. These schemas are formed in childhood and adolescence and develop through adulthood. EMSs are maintained because they filter new experiences, both internal and external, and distort their meaning to confirm the EMS. EMS responses may have been adaptive earlier in life (e.g., the coping modes are versions of fight, flight, or freeze survival responses), but by adulthood they are maladaptive and interfere with people getting their needs met. EMSs become unhealthy core beliefs and rules that a person wholeheartedly accepts. EMSs, while dormant, are easily accessed when activated by internal (implicit memory and the sensory system) or external cues (e.g., interactions with others, certain sights, sounds, smells).

Schema modes were defined by Young et al. (2003) as "the current emotional, cognitive, behavioral, and neurobiological state that a person experiences" (p. 43). They can be viewed as parts of self that are triggered when EMSs are activated. Young et al. described four types of modes: healthy adult modes, demanding/punitive inner critic modes, maladaptive coping modes, and innate child modes. These are described in Appendix C.

The Goals of Schema Therapy in Mode Terms

This book presents 12 core skills of ST. It is important to consider the relevance of these skills in achieving the treatment goals of ST. The primary goal is to build up and fortify the healthy adult mode to enable a person to have an emotionally healthy and happy life. Strengthening the healthy adult mode means that the individual gains greater access to mindful and empathic awareness, caring and thoughtful decision making, and adaptive skills when dysfunctional modes are triggered. In the early stages of ST, these are the goals of the therapist, which are seen as part of limited reparenting. In the autonomy stage, these become the goals of the client's healthy adult mode.

1. Care for the vulnerable child mode. This is a function of the internal "good parent" part of the healthy adult mode.

2. Develop awareness of the maladaptive coping modes to be able to choose more effective responses that meet the present need without negative results.

3. Understand and channel angry or impulsive/undisciplined child mode reactions into assertive and effective ways to get needs met.

4. Reduce the power and control of the demanding/punitive inner critic mode and develop ways to motivate oneself positively, accepting mistakes as part of the learning process and taking responsibility for them. This includes setting reasonable expectancies and standards.

5. Be able to evoke the happy child mode to be able to embrace opportunities for joy and play.

6. Be able to access the competence of the healthy adult mode.

The Stages of Schema Therapy

The course of ST generally has three stages: bonding and emotional regulation, mode change, and autonomy (Young et al., 2003). The order of these stages will vary, determined by the individual client and therapist. Table 1.2 presents the relationship between the stages of ST, the four main components of ST (described in the next section), and the ST deliberate practice skills from Table 1.1.

The Four Main Components of Schema Therapy Interventions

Limited Reparenting

Limited reparenting (LRP) is both the therapist's role and a treatment intervention. LRP is thought to be an integral part of the change process in ST. It provides corrective emotional experiences, which are essential to heal EMS and provide a base in the experience of having needs met. This base allows the formation of more positive and adaptive core beliefs. In LRP, the therapist models making active choices of healthy and adaptive behaviors to reduce the use of maladaptive coping mode behavior. LRP provides "good parent" responses and messages to reduce the power of the demanding/ punitive inner critic modes. In summary, a schema therapist meets the client's needs like a good parent would, bounded by the ethical limits of therapy. In the LRP role, the schema therapist provides safety, understanding, and comfort for the vulnerable child mode; listens to and acknowledges the needs of the angry child; and confronts and sets healthy limits for the impulsive or undisciplined child mode. Clients in the vulnerable child mode need a "good parent" therapist to use the words and tone of a parent talking to a young child who is lonely, frightened, sad, and so forth. Schema therapists become firm and resolute advocates for the vulnerable child, identifying and confronting maladaptive coping modes or inner critic modes, empathizing with the feelings and needs underneath the mode while challenging whether the action taken is effective. Clients with personality disorders or complex trauma require this active reparenting in the early phase of treatment because they are frequently in child modes and have an underdeveloped healthy adult mode.

TABLE 1.2. The 12 Skills in Relation to the Stages of Schema Therapy

Schema Therapy Component	Deliberate Practice Skill
Bonding and emotional regulation	
Limited reparenting	Skill 1. Understanding and attunement
	Skill 3. Schema education: beginning to understand current problems in schema therapy terms
	Skill 4. Linking unmet needs, schema, and presenting problem
Mode change	
Mode awareness	Skill 5. Education about maladaptive schema modes
	Skill 6. Recognizing the mode shifts of the maladaptive coping modes
	Skill 7. Identifying the presence of the demanding/punitive inner critic mode
	Skill 8. Identifying the presence of the angry and vulnerable child modes
Limited reparenting, mode healing	Skill 9. Limited reparenting for the angry and vulnerable child modes
	Skill 10. Limited reparenting for the demanding/punitive inner critic mode
	Skill 11. Limited reparenting for the maladaptive coping modes: empathic confrontation
Autonomy	
Mode management	Skill 2. Supporting and strengthening the healthy adult mode
	Skill 12. Implementing behavioral pattern breaking through homework assignments

Note. The gray rows represent the three stages of schema therapy. Each stage contains one or more of the four components of schema therapy: limited reparenting, mode awareness, mode healing, and mode management.

As the client's healthy modes develop, the therapist shifts, becoming poised in the role of a healthy reparenting agent for an adolescent or a healthy model for the developing adult. Clients will still need connection with the therapist in the later phase of treatment, but they can do most of their own "reparenting" from what they have internalized into their further developed and fortified healthy adult (Younan et al., 2018). Schema therapists are keen to recognize that the strategies, including use of language, level of sophistication, and timing/pacing of strategy application must take into account and be consistent with the client's developmental capacities, comorbidity challenges, and any at-risk issues.

Limited and adaptive reparenting starts with a robust assessment and schema conceptualization that inform treatment goals and strategies. The therapist is poised in an active, supportive, and authentic relationship with the client, one that offers safe connection and a human realness devoid of therapeutic jargon and hierarchical posture. The client is welcome to express vulnerability—emotions and needs. The therapy relationship, albeit limited, fills critical needs–meeting gaps through modeling and mirroring and reimagined ways of experiencing oneself securely attached; ideally, the client feels valued and worthy, often for the first time. Initially, the therapist provides frequent and emphasized reassurance regarding the client's value, security, stability, safety, acceptance, empathy, support, advocacy, and identity. The therapy relationship supports clients learning to meet their needs effectively, improving interpersonal skills and attaining autonomy while being able to maintain healthy connection. The ST approach to meeting needs within professional boundaries is quite different than the approach of most other therapy models, which assume more healthy adult mode and skills than clients have and focus too early on clients meeting their own needs when they have never had the experience of them being met. Exercises 1, 2, 3, 4, 9, 10, and 11 in this volume all include aspects of limited reparenting.

Mode Awareness

Mode awareness is usually the first step in the mode change stage of treatment. These interventions are primarily cognitive. Mode awareness work teaches the client to notice when a mode is triggered, identify the underlying schema activated, and the present need (see Appendix C for more details about the relationship between schema mode experiences and underlying, unmet needs). Clients become able to identify their thoughts, feelings, physical sensations, and memories when a mode is present. They learn to connect their reactions in the present to childhood experiences upon which EMS and modes have formed. When clients connect their current situation to childhood memories, they better understand the roots of their schemas and modes (Farrell et al., 2014). Mode awareness is necessary for a client to make a deliberate choice whether to allow a mode to continue or to connect with their healthy adult mode and their skills. Exercises 6, 7, and 8 focus on the mood awareness component of ST.

Mode Management

Mode management skills make use of mode awareness to choose more effective responses. Mode awareness must be present for mode change, but it is not sufficient. The client and therapist evaluate whether the maladaptive mode response will meet their present need or if a different action will be more effective. In mode management work, an alternate, more effective plan to meet the need is developed and implemented. The mode management component of ST includes cognitive, behavioral, and experiential techniques. The therapist identifies and challenges the client's barriers to change, such as actions, cognitive distortions, or beliefs that maintain maladaptive mode behavior. Mode management plans are a powerful method for taking the behavioral-pattern-breaking work of ST out of the therapy room and into the client's daily life (Farrell et al., 2018). There are elements of the mode management component in Exercises 2 and 12. In general, much of this work is in the third stage of ST.

Mode Healing

Mode healing involves experiential mode work, which begins with the corrective emotional experiences of the therapy relationship (e.g., limited reparenting), then goes on to include visual imagery, imagery rescripting, mode dialogues, mode role-plays, and creative work to symbolize positive experiences. These ST interventions are designed to reach deep into the emotional and somatic levels of awareness, targeting early experiences and rescripting experiences that can lead to sustainable levels of change. The skills in Exercises 9, 10, and 11 are part of the mode healing component. Methods for mode healing can be creative and symbolic, such as using art or written material to facilitate the client's recall and the emotional reexperiencing of schema-contradicting events (Farrell et al., 2014).

The Schema Therapy Case Conceptualization

ST is guided by a comprehensive case conceptualization, which guides the work and identifies the client's schemas, modes, and unmet needs. The ST Case Conceptualization (downloadable at https://schematherapysociety.org) offers a mutually agreed-upon assessment between therapist and client about how current life challenges and lack of satisfaction may be linked with schemas and modes, providing a therapeutic road map for both formulating and navigating a thoughtful treatment plan. The ST conceptualization also includes the therapist's appraisal of the therapy relationship, including an appreciation for the parallel process of therapist/client moment-to-moment, in-session observations and behavioral responses and the therapist's personal feelings about the client. Each skill in this book targets a schema or mode, often both, and is designed as a step in accomplishing one of the treatment objectives for the given client. For an overview of some major ST concepts, see Appendix C.

The Evidence Base of Schema Therapy

The evidence base for the effectiveness of ST includes several large randomized controlled trials of individual and group ST for borderline, avoidant, and dependent personality disorders; posttraumatic stress disorder; complex trauma; dissociative identity disorder; eating disorders; and chronic depression (summarized in Farrell & Shaw, 2022). The effectiveness of ST reported in these studies includes decreases in psychiatric symptoms, as well as improved function and quality of life. Clients and therapists were found to prefer ST methods to those of other models in qualitative studies (de Klerk et al., 2017).

The Role of Deliberate Practice in Schema Therapy Training

ST training already includes a significant amount of dyadic practice. Fifteen of the 40 hours of basic training required for international certification in ST must be dyadic. The importance of clinical skills practice was given empirical support by a study that investigated the role of practice in producing effective schema therapists. Bamelis et al. (2014) found that therapists trained with a practice focus (e.g., role-playing of specific techniques with immediate feedback) were better equipped to apply techniques with real clients than those who only followed lecture-based training.

We believe that the approach of deliberate practice, which includes identifying core microskills, encouraging practitioners to monitor their client outcomes, and a practice system designed to keep therapists in the zone of proximal development, is consistent with the training approach of ST and should improve our current training programs. The goal of deliberate practice to support therapists in making skills their own is consistent with the genuineness and flexibility that effective ST requires.

A Note About Vocal Tone and Body Posture

ST training emphasizes the need to attend to the nonverbal and paralinguistic cues expressed by both client and therapist. Effective ST involves the therapist's careful, moment-by-moment reading of the client's communication as expressed verbally and nonverbally. The therapist in turn is trained to be aware of their own tone of voice, facial expression, and body posture to convey the attitudes of warmth, empathy, genuine curiosity, and openness through their moment-by-moment responding. For each one of the ST skills covered in this book, therapists should be mindful of attending to and practicing their nonverbal interpersonal qualities, such as tone of voice and body posture. It is additionally useful for ST learners to watch recorded examples of ST experts performing therapy so that they can observe these key principles in action.

Overview of the Book's Structure

This book is organized into three parts. Part I contains this chapter and Chapter 2, which provides basic instructions on how to perform these exercises. We found through testing that providing too many instructions up front overwhelmed trainers and trainees, and they skipped past them as a result. Therefore, we kept these instructions as brief and simple as possible to focus only on the most essential information that trainers and trainees will need to get started with the exercises. Further guidelines for getting the most out of deliberate practice are provided in Chapter 3, and additional instructions for monitoring and adjusting the difficulty of the exercises are provided in Appendix A. **Do not skip the instructions in Chapter 2, and be sure to read the additional guidelines and instructions in Chapter 3 and Appendix A once you are comfortable with the basic instructions.**

Part II contains the 12 skill-focused exercises, which are ordered based on their difficulty: beginner, intermediate, and advanced (see Table 1.1). They each contain a brief overview of the exercise, example client–therapist interactions to help guide trainees, step-by-step instructions for conducting that exercise, and a list of criteria for mastering the relevant skill. The client statements and sample therapist responses are then presented, also organized by difficulty (beginner, intermediate, and advanced). The statements and responses are presented separately so that the trainee playing the therapist has more freedom to improvise responses without being influenced by the sample responses, which should only be turned to if the trainee has difficulty improvising their own responses. The last two exercises in Part II provide opportunities to practice the 12 skills within simulated psychotherapy sessions. Exercise 13 provides a sample psychotherapy session transcript in which the ST skills are used and clearly labeled, thereby demonstrating how they might flow together in an actual therapy session. Trainees are invited to run through the sample transcript with one playing the therapist and the other playing the client to get a feel for how a session might unfold. Exercise 14 provides suggestions for undertaking mock sessions, as well as client profiles ordered by difficulty (beginner, intermediate, and advanced) that trainees can use for improvised role-plays.

Part III contains Chapter 3, which provides additional guidance for trainers and trainees. While Chapter 2 is more procedural, Chapter 3 covers big-picture issues. It highlights six key points for getting the most out of deliberate practice and describes the importance of appropriate responsiveness, attending to trainee well-being and respecting their privacy, and trainer self-evaluation, among other topics.

Four appendixes conclude this book. Appendix A provides instructions for monitoring and adjusting the difficulty of each exercise as needed. It provides a Deliberate Practice Reaction Form for the trainee playing the therapist to complete to indicate whether the exercise is too easy or too difficult. Appendix B includes a Deliberate Practice Diary Form, which provides a format for trainees to explore and record their experiences while engaging in deliberate practice. Appendix C contains a review of key concepts in ST that trainees can study to guide their practice when performing the exercises in this book. Appendix D presents a sample syllabus demonstrating how the 14 deliberate practice exercises and other support material can be integrated into a wider ST training course. Instructors may choose to modify the syllabus or pick elements of it to integrate into their own courses.

Downloadable versions of this book's appendixes, including a color version of the Deliberate Practice Reaction Form, can be found in the "Clinician and Practitioner Resources" tab online (https://www.apa.org/pubs/books/deliberate-practice-schema-therapy).

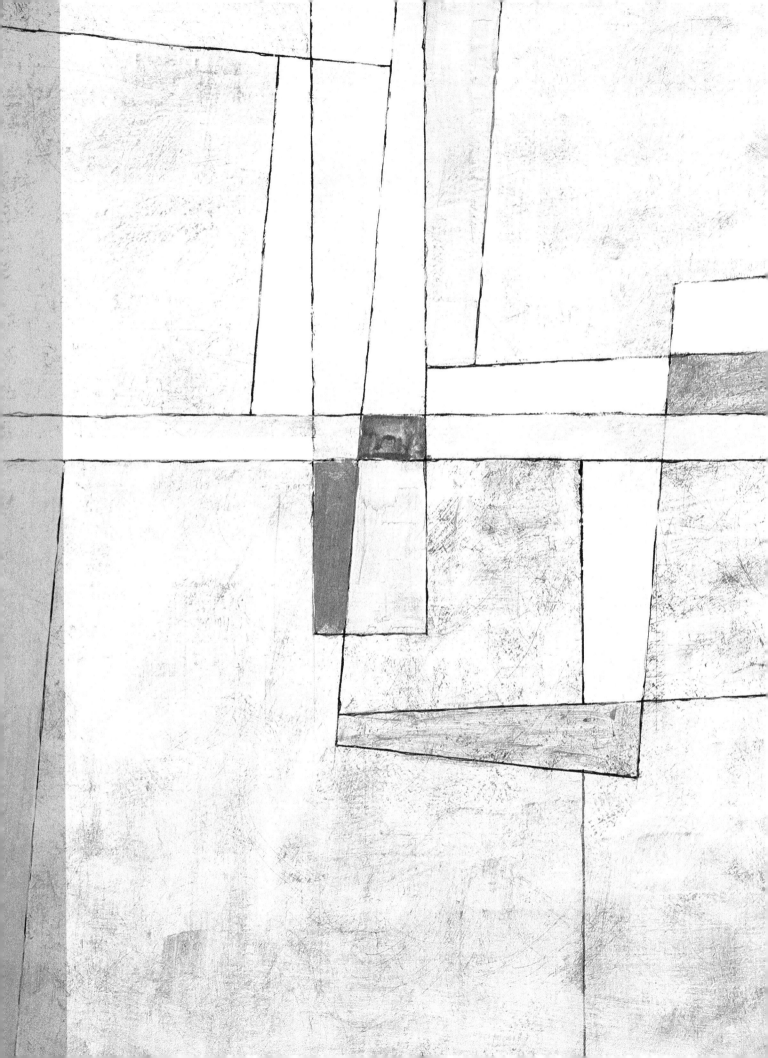

Instructions for the Schema Therapy Deliberate Practice Exercises

This chapter provides basic instructions that are common to all the exercises in this book. More specific instructions are provided in each exercise. Chapter 3 also provides important guidance for trainees and trainers that will help them get the most out of deliberate practice. Appendix A offers additional instructions for monitoring and adjusting the difficulty of the exercises as needed after getting through all then client statements in a single difficulty level, including a Deliberate Practice Reaction Form the trainee playing the therapist can complete to indicate whether they found the statements too easy or too difficult. **Difficulty assessment is an important part of the deliberate practice process and should not be skipped.**

Overview

The deliberate practice exercises in this book involve role-plays of hypothetical situations in therapy. The role-play involves three people: One trainee role-plays the therapist, another trainee role-plays the client, and a trainer (professor/supervisor) observes and provides feedback. Alternately, a peer can observe and provide feedback.

This book provides a script for each role-play, each with a client statement and also with an example therapist response. The client statements are graded in difficulty from beginning to advanced, although these difficulty grades are only estimates. The actual perceived difficulty of client statements is subjective and varies widely by trainee. For example, some trainees may experience a stimulus of a client being angry as easy to respond to, whereas another trainee may experience it as very difficult. Thus, it is important for trainees to provide difficulty assessments and adjustments to ensure that they are practicing at the right difficulty level: neither too easy nor too hard.

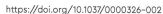

https://doi.org/10.1037/0000326-002

Deliberate Practice in Schema Therapy, by W. T. Behary, J. M. Farrell, A. Vaz, and T. Rousmaniere

Time Frame

We recommend a 90-minute time block for every exercise, structured roughly as follows:

- First 20 minutes: Orientation—the trainer explains the schema therapy skill and demonstrates the exercise procedure with a volunteer trainee.

- Middle 50 minutes: Trainees perform the exercise in pairs. The trainer or a peer provides feedback throughout this process and monitors or adjusts the exercise's difficulty as needed after each set of statements (see Appendix A for more information about difficulty assessment).

- Final 20 minutes: Review, feedback, and discussion.

Preparation

1. Every trainee will need their own copy of this book.

2. Each exercise requires the trainer to fill out a Deliberate Practice Reaction Form after completing all the statements from a single difficulty level. This form is available in the "Clinician and Practitioner Resources" tab at https://www.apa.org/pubs/books/deliberate-practice-schema-therapy and in Appendix A.

3. Trainees are grouped into pairs. One volunteers to role-play the therapist and one to role-play the client (they will switch roles after 15 minutes of practice). As noted previously, an observer who might be either the trainer or a fellow trainee will work with each pair.

The Role of the Trainer

The primary responsibilities of the trainer are to

1. provide corrective feedback, which includes both information about how well the trainees' response met expected criteria and any necessary guidance about how to improve the response, and

2. remind trainees to do difficulty assessments and adjustments after each level of client statements is completed (beginning, intermediate, and advanced).

How to Practice

Each exercise includes its own step-by-step instructions. Trainees should follow these instructions carefully, as every step is important.

Skill Criteria

Each of the first 12 exercises focuses on one essential schema therapy skill with two to four skill criteria that describe the important components or principles for that skill.

The goal of the role-play is for trainees to practice improvising responses to the client statement in a manner that (a) is attuned to the client, (b) meets skill criteria as much as possible, and (c) feels authentic for the trainee. Trainees are provided scripts with example therapist responses to give them a sense of how to incorporate the skill criteria into a response. **It is important, however, that trainees do not read the example responses verbatim in the role-plays!** Therapy is highly personal and improvisational; the goal of deliberate practice is to develop trainees' ability to improvise within a consistent framework. Memorizing scripted responses would be counterproductive for helping trainees learn to perform therapy that is responsive, authentic, and attuned to each individual client.

Wendy Behary and Joan Farrell wrote the scripted example responses. However, trainees' personal style of therapy may differ slightly or significantly from that in the example scripts. It is essential that, over time, trainees develop their own style and voice, while simultaneously being able to intervene according to the model's principles and strategies. To facilitate this, the exercises in this book were designed to maximize opportunities for improvisational responses informed by the skill criteria and ongoing feedback. Trainees will note that some of the scripted responses do not meet all the skill criteria: These responses are provided as examples of flexible application of schema therapy skills in a manner that prioritizes attunement with the client.

Review, Feedback, and Discussion

The review and feedback sequence after each role-play has these two elements:

- First, the trainee who played the client **briefly** shares how it felt to be on the receiving end of the therapist response. This can help assess how well trainees are attuning with the client.

- Second, the trainer provides **brief** feedback (less than 1 minute) based on the skill criteria for each exercise. Keep feedback specific, behavioral, and brief to preserve time for skill rehearsal. If one trainer is teaching multiple pairs of trainees, the trainer walks around room, observing the pairs and offering brief feedback. When the trainer is not available, the trainee playing the client gives peer feedback to the therapist, based on the skill criteria and how it felt to be on the receiving end of the intervention. Alternatively, a third trainee can observe and provide feedback.

Trainers (or peers) should remember to keep all feedback specific and brief and not to veer into discussions of theory. There are many other settings for extended discussion of schema therapy theory and research. In deliberate practice, it is of utmost importance to maximize time for continuous behavioral rehearsal via role-plays.

Final Evaluation

After both trainees have role-played the client and the therapist, the trainer provides an evaluation. Participants should engage in a short group discussion based on this evaluation. This discussion can provide ideas for where to focus homework and future deliberate practice sessions. To this end, Appendix B presents a Deliberate Practice Diary Form, which can also be downloaded from the "Clinician and Practitioner Resources" tab online (https://www.apa.org/pubs/books/deliberate-practice-schema-therapy). This form can be used as part of the final evaluation to help trainees process their experiences from that session with the supervisor. However, it is designed primarily to be used by trainees as a template for exploring and recording their thoughts and experiences between sessions, particularly when pursuing additional deliberate practice activities without the supervisor, such as rehearsing responses alone or if two trainees want to practice the exercises together—perhaps with a third trainee filling the supervisor's role. Then, if they want, the trainees can discuss these experiences with the supervisor at the beginning of the next training session.

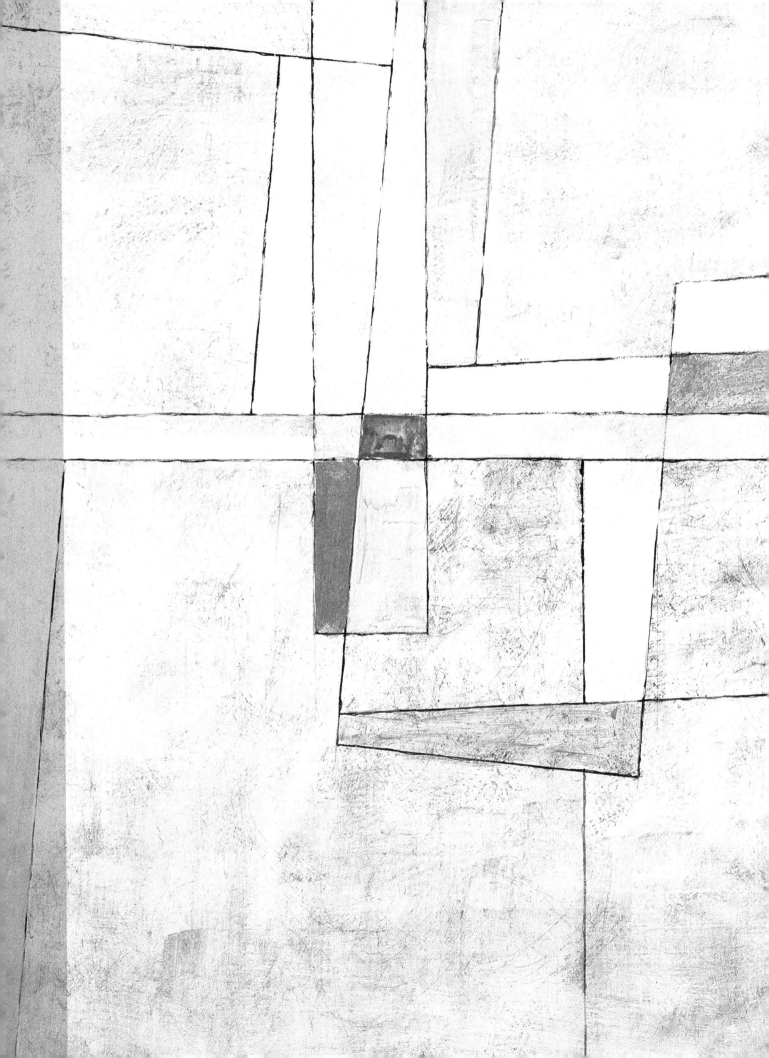

Deliberate Practice Exercises for Schema Therapy Skills

This section of the book provides 12 deliberate practice exercises for essential schema therapy (ST) skills. These exercises are organized in a developmental sequence, from those that are more appropriate to someone just beginning ST training to those who have progressed to a more advanced level. Although we anticipate that most trainers would use these exercises in the order we have suggested, some may find it more appropriate to their training circumstances to use a different order. We also provide two comprehensive exercises that bring together the ST skills using an annotated ST session transcript and mock ST sessions.

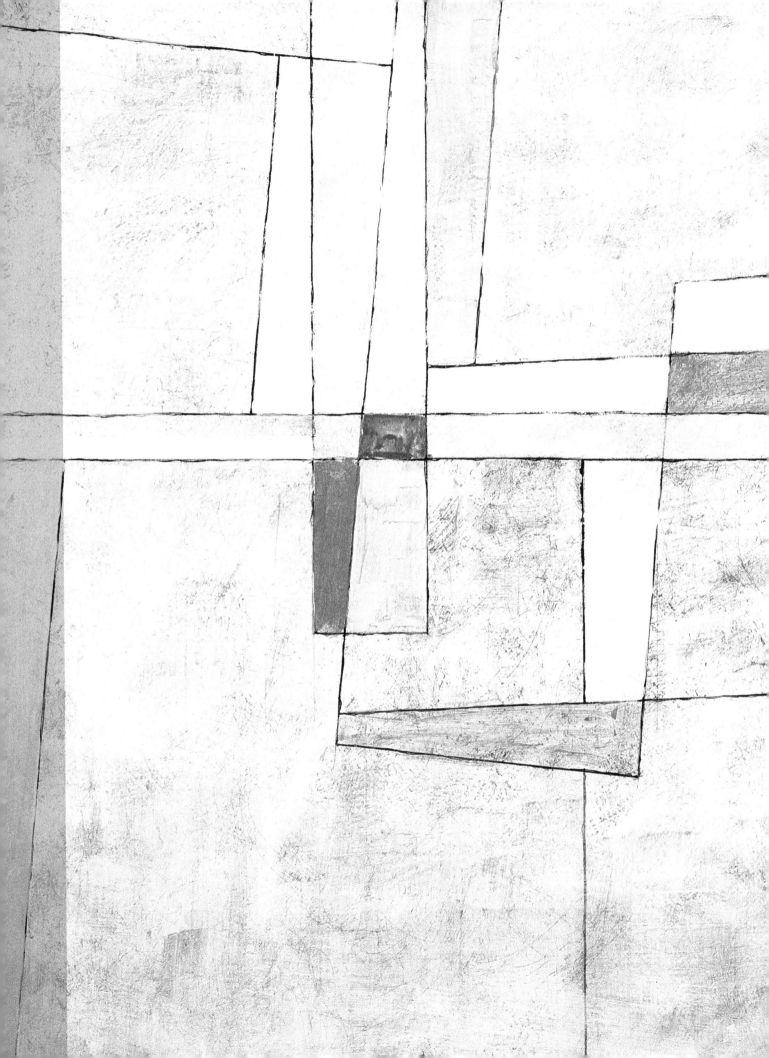

Understanding and Attunement

Preparations for Exercise 1

1. Read the instructions in Chapter 2.

2. Download the Deliberate Practice Reaction Form and Deliberate Practice Diary Form at https://www.apa.org/pubs/books/deliberate-practice-schema-therapy (see the "Clinician and Practitioner Resources" tab; also available in Appendixes A and B, respectively).

Skill Description

Skill Difficulty Level: Beginner

The therapist's attunement and demonstrated interest in understanding the experiences of the client are central to forging the necessary bond for connection and trust. Creating a trusting bond with clients is essential for the therapeutic alliance and for the corrective relational experience of limited reparenting, which is essential for schema therapy. There are many methods schema therapists use to facilitate a safe bond with clients. We focus here on understanding and attunement, a method widely used throughout therapy (Bailey & Ogles, 2019).

For this exercise, the therapist should improvise a response to each client statement following these skill criteria:

1. The therapist's ability to attune and empathize is communicated in their expressed understanding of the client's "internal reality," as reflected by both what the client explicitly says and what the client communicates in nonverbal ways. The therapist starts their interventions by reflecting the core meanings or feelings communicated by the client. They may also express validation for the content (e.g., "What you are sharing is really important").

2. After communicating understanding of the client, the therapist reassures them by expressing their desire to be helpful, to want to make sure they feel safe, or by making

https://doi.org/10.1037/0000326-003

Deliberate Practice in Schema Therapy, by W. T. Behary, J. M. Farrell, A. Vaz, and T. Rousmaniere

invitations to collaborate in therapy. This reassurance is often a new relational experience for many clients and as such should be valued.

3. Throughout this exercise, the therapist's nonverbal tone and body position convey openness and warmth toward the client. This criterion is crucial because therapists' nonverbals are essential to communicate attunement and facilitate safety with clients.

SKILL CRITERIA FOR EXERCISE 1

1. Communicate an empathic understanding of the client's "internal reality."
2. Reassure the client about your desire to understand and be helpful to them.
3. Nonverbal: Use a soft, warm voice and slight movement toward the client.

Examples of Understanding and Attunement

Example 1

CLIENT: [*Nervous*] I just don't know what to say. I have never told anyone about my personal feelings or my life story. How do I start? I am not sure this was a good decision to go to therapy. I know my mother would be so furious with me if she knew.

THERAPIST: It's a very big decision to start therapy—to share your life experiences, your struggles, and your strengths with a stranger. (Criterion 1) It will take a little time to feel secure and confident in this relationship with me, and I want to make sure you feel safe and trusting in my care. This is your private space, and your mother need not know about your decision to come to therapy. (Criterion 2)

Example 2

CLIENT: [*Flat*] I just don't want you to think I am a pathetic loser, which is the only thing you could think once you get to know me. Well, maybe it will give you a laugh or something amusing to share with your therapist friends when you hear my story. Or maybe you will get bored like my last therapist and be sorry you ever agreed to work with me.

THERAPIST: I am sorry to hear that your last experience was disappointing for you. Starting therapy is a big decision and not easy. I am glad to meet you and look forward to getting to know you. (Criterion 1) Is there anything that I might say or do that could help you to feel safer in this relationship? Perhaps regarding the privacy of these meetings, or about my thoughts and feelings as you share your experiences and needs with me? It is important to me that you feel respected in this space. (Criterion 2)

Example 3

CLIENT: [*Anxious*] I know it's just a 50-minute session and I will probably need a thousand sessions, but I have to get this off my chest right away. So, I was coming from the lunchroom at work when I get approached by my supervisor, who immediately gives me the look like I am in trouble, and before she could say anything, I started to cry and made a complete fool of myself. I hate my job. I can't do anything right! Oh wow, I am just going on and on. Are you sure you want to work with me?

THERAPIST: You have a lot to share and that's okay. The early days of therapy can be hard for figuring out how best to identify goals and share experiences. (Criterion 1) I will help you with that. You don't ever need to apologize for sharing your experiences. I will help you make sure that the information and the feelings you share with me are consistent with meeting your needs. (Criterion 2)

INSTRUCTIONS FOR EXERCISE 1

Step 1: Role-Play and Feedback

- The client says the first beginner client statement. The therapist improvises a response based on the skill criteria.
- The trainer (or, if not available, the client) provides brief feedback based on the skill criteria.
- The client then repeats the same statement, and the therapist again improvises a response. The trainer (or client) again provides brief feedback.

Step 2: Repeat

- Repeat Step 1 for all the statements in the current difficulty level (beginner, intermediate, or advanced).

Step 3: Assess and Adjust Difficulty

- The therapist completes the Deliberate Practice Reaction Form (see Appendix A) and decides whether to make the exercise easier or harder or to repeat the same difficulty level.

Step 4: Repeat for Approximately 15 Minutes

- Repeat Steps 1 to 3 for at least 15 minutes.
- The trainees then switch therapist and client roles and start over.

Now it's your turn! Follow Steps 1 and 2 from the instructions.

Remember: The goal of the role-play is for trainees to practice improvising responses to the client statements in a manner that (a) uses the skill criteria and (b) feels authentic for the trainee. **Example therapist responses for each client statement are provided at the end of this exercise. Trainees should attempt to improvise their own responses before reading the example responses.**

BEGINNER-LEVEL CLIENT STATEMENTS FOR EXERCISE 1
Beginner Client Statement 1
[Hesitant] Where do I start? I've never done this therapy thing before, and I don't want to get it wrong on my first try and look stupid.
Beginner Client Statement 2
[Shaky] Oh, this is so silly. I don't know why I am already wanting to cry. I haven't even told you anything yet. This is so embarrassing.
Beginner Client Statement 3
[Sad] I don't think I can change. I mean, I know my anger is a problem, and I don't mean to be hurtful to my partner. But I just don't feel hopeful about changing my reactions when I get upset, and that means I am going to lose my relationship.
Beginner Client Statement 4
[Nervous] I don't know how I'm going to tell my whole story in a 50-minute therapy session! I feel like I have so much to tell you. You need to have a very clear picture . . . and I know you probably think this is crazy, but I have to tell you everything!
Beginner Client Statement 5
[Sad] I just feel sad today. I don't have any energy. How do you keep going when you have bad days? I forgot you probably can't answer that. Sorry, forget that I asked it.

 Assess and adjust the difficulty before moving to the next difficulty level (see Step 3 in the exercise instructions).

INTERMEDIATE-LEVEL CLIENT STATEMENTS FOR EXERCISE 1

Intermediate Client Statement 1

[Confused] I don't know what to think. My father always said I shouldn't aim too high, but you are saying that I should pay attention to what I really want to do. I want to go to medical school, and I have the grades for it, according to my college counselor.

Intermediate Client Statement 2

[Anxious] What should I do about asking my boyfriend to marry me? He is like my knight in shining armor most of the time, but sometimes he is cold and withdraws and I can't reach him for days. There is such a big contrast in his behavior. But I don't want to lose him if he is "the one." I am close to a panic attack.

Intermediate Client Statement 3

[Agitated] I don't want to talk about anything heavy like last session. I have an important negotiation meeting to attend right after this and I need to be sharp and at my best, not musing about my childhood experiences.

Intermediate Client Statement 4

[Looking down] I wasn't going to come to session today. You must be so tired of listening to me complaining and not doing what I need to do. I am not even sure why I came in. I just want to go home and order a pizza.

Intermediate Client Statement 5

[Scared] I think if you really knew me, I mean if you knew everything about me, you would be disgusted. I just don't know how anyone could ever really accept me after all the shameful failures I've had in my life.

 Assess and adjust the difficulty before moving to the next difficulty level (see Step 3 in the exercise instructions).

ADVANCED-LEVEL CLIENT STATEMENTS FOR EXERCISE 1
Advanced Client Statement 1
[Sad] I just don't think anything will ever change. I didn't get my emotional needs met as a child and now you are telling me that I have to learn to meet them for myself.
Advanced Client Statement 2
[Anxious] I don't know what to think. You told me that I have a right to express my feelings, but when I do, my wife gets really mad at me. I am really rocking the boat and it's scary.
Advanced Client Statement 3
[Confused] I'm very angry with my best friend for sharing personal information of mine with her wife. She told me that she was trying to get some feedback to help me because her wife is a doctor, but I feel so betrayed. This feels crazy to be so torn.
Advanced Client Statement 4
[Frustrated] I just don't want to be here today. I am tired of focusing on myself and my petty grievances. There are people in the world with real problems—not whiny, neurotic complaints like mine.
Advanced Client Statement 5
[Irritated] I want to make sure today that we have time to discuss my agenda. I think that you choose what we focus on too often. I know that you are the expert. I probably shouldn't be saying any of this. I should just go along with what you think is best.

🛑 **Assess and adjust the difficulty here (see Step 3 in the exercise instructions). If appropriate, follow the instructions to make the exercise even more challenging (see Appendix A).**

Example Therapist Responses: Understanding and Attunement

Remember: Trainees should attempt to improvise their own responses before reading the example responses. **Do not read the following responses verbatim unless you are having trouble coming up with your own responses!**

EXAMPLE RESPONSES TO BEGINNER-LEVEL CLIENT STATEMENTS FOR EXERCISE 1
Example Response to Beginner Client Statement 1
I hear that you are a bit anxious about trying therapy, where you don't know what is expected and don't want to make a bad first impression. (Criterion 1) It is okay to start anywhere. You aren't in this alone. I am here to help you. I am happy to make a suggestion about where we might start today. (Criterion 2)
Example Response to Beginner Client Statement 2
Oh, it's not silly at all. I can imagine that perhaps as you anticipate sharing your pain, it's upsetting and maybe even a little scary? (Criterion 1) All feelings are welcome here. (Criterion 2)
Example Response to Beginner Client Statement 3
I can appreciate your worries about losing your relationship, given that you feel hopeless about your capacity to change this behavior. (Criterion 1) Once we see what's driving this reaction, I will help you to learn how to bypass it and develop healthier responses. (Criterion 2)
Example Response to Beginner Client Statement 4
Okay, let's take a breath together. I can see that you have a lot to share with me. I don't think this is crazy at all. Just take your time. (Criterion 1) I can't wait to get to know you, and we will have plenty of time in the coming weeks to make that happen. (Criterion 2)
Example Response to Beginner Client Statement 5
You don't have to apologize, and it is okay to ask me questions. I am glad that you got here today even with no energy. (Criterion 1) I want to understand your sadness and the needs that underlie it. Yes, I have bad days too, and I can help you work with yours. (Criterion 2)

EXAMPLE RESPONSES TO INTERMEDIATE-LEVEL CLIENT STATEMENTS FOR EXERCISE 1

Example Response to Intermediate Client Statement 1

I understand that this would be confusing for you. Your father discouraged you from aiming too high, and I have tried to help you consider your dreams. Your counselor is looking at the hard evidence. (Criterion 1) Would it help for us to look at these three positions together? (Criterion 2)

Example Response to Intermediate Client Statement 2

Wow! What a lot of pressure and confusion you are feeling! Those are very different sets of behavior from one person. This is a really important decision to make. (Criterion 1) Why don't you take a deep breath, and we can look at the pros and cons together. Would that be helpful for you? (Criterion 2)

Example Response to Intermediate Client Statement 3

I understand that it feels difficult to reconcile such an important meeting coming after our work together. The pressure has led to you being dismissive about the importance of your childhood experiences. (Criterion 1) I want to do what will be most helpful for you today. That might be reminding you of your business competence. What do you think? (Criterion 2)

Example Response to Intermediate Client Statement 4

I know it's hard for you to imagine that someone might really care for you, even when you are struggling and not achieving. (Criterion 1) But this is me, and I care about you. We are going to get through this. I am so glad you decided to come in today. (Criterion 2)

Example Response to Intermediate Client Statement 5

It's always scary sharing all the parts of ourselves with someone. Of course, it feels risky given all the deprivation and rejection you suffered in your childhood. (Criterion 1) I really do want to know you and cannot imagine feeling disgust. I care about you and your wellness. (Criterion 2)

EXAMPLE RESPONSES TO ADVANCED-LEVEL CLIENT STATEMENTS FOR EXERCISE 1

Example Response to Advanced Client Statement 1

It is difficult for you not to feel hopeless since you have had so little experience of having your needs met when you were a child, or by anyone now. That would make it very hard when you think you are hearing that no one will meet your needs now either. (Criterion 1) Fortunately, that is not my message to you. I will help you get your needs met in our sessions. You are not alone in this. (Criterion 2)

Example Response to Advanced Client Statement 2

It must be confusing to think that you are doing what is healthy and it gets a negative response. You might even feel a little angry at me about how that worked out. (Criterion 1) I want you to know that you have my support in this and I know it is difficult. Let's look together at the details of what happened and see what comes next. (Criterion 2)

Example Response to Advanced Client Statement 3

I hear that it is very confusing to have such strong, conflicted feelings. You love your friend and believe that she had good intentions, but you also feel betrayed. (Criterion 1) Let's talk some more about all that you feel about your friend and this situation to have the big picture. (Criterion 2)

Example Response to Advanced Client Statement 4

It is difficult for you to take your problems and pain seriously because you compare them to the worst-case scenario in the world. When you do that, it is difficult for you to feel they are important. You may also worry about whether I think they are important. (Criterion 1) I know they are, and I want to reassure you that I understand your dilemma and want to look at your complaints. (Criterion 2)

Example Response to Advanced Client Statement 5

So, you are feeling that there is not a balance here in terms of who sets our agenda and even worry about whether it is okay to tell me this. (Criterion 1) I am sorry that you are left feeling that it is not okay for you to take the lead here. This is your time, and there is always room for topics you want on the agenda. Why don't we set the agenda together before we start our sessions? (Criterion 2)

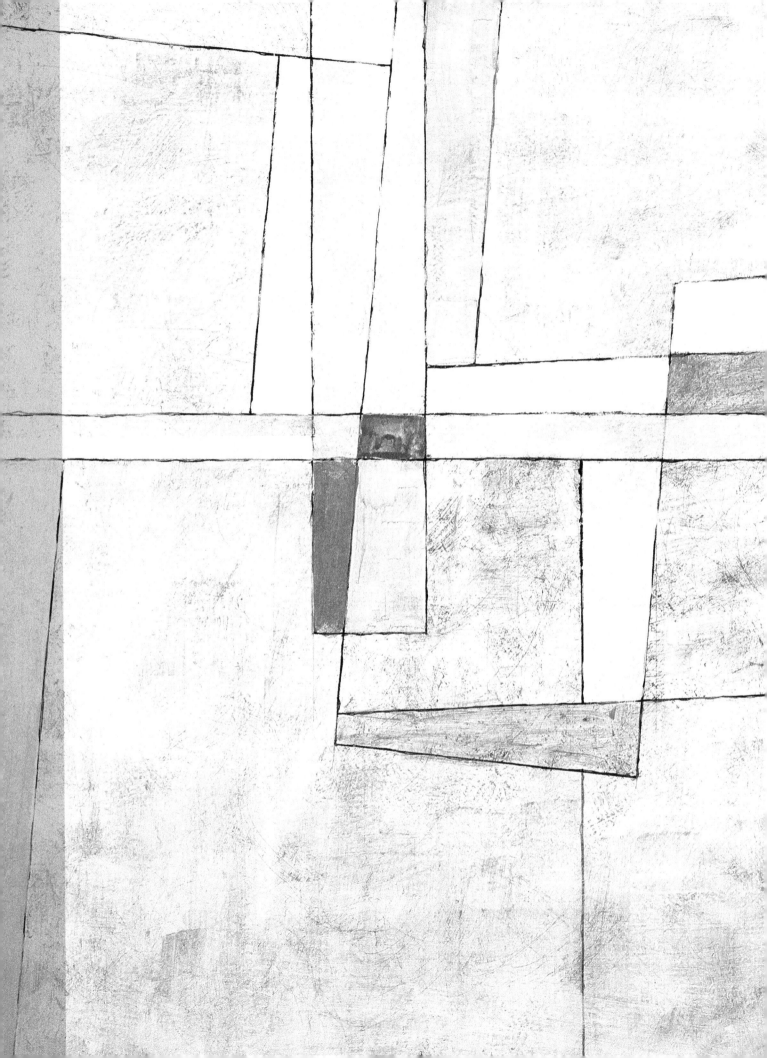

Supporting and Strengthening the Healthy Adult Mode

Preparations for Exercise 2

1. Read the instructions in Chapter 2.

2. Download the Deliberate Practice Reaction Form and Deliberate Practice Diary Form at https://www.apa.org/pubs/books/deliberate-practice-schema-therapy (see the "Clinician and Practitioner Resources" tab; also available in Appendixes A and B, respectively).

Skill Description

Skill Difficulty Level: Beginner

Supporting and strengthening the healthy adult mode in schema therapy consists of acknowledging the client's autonomy, competence, and internalization of a loving and nurturing inner caregiver. The healthy adult mode is conceptualized as the rational, warm, and competent adult part of all of us that nurtures, protects, and validates the vulnerable child part; sets limits for the angry and impulsive child parts; promotes and supports the happy child; confronts and eventually replaces the unhealthy coping modes with adaptive ones; and neutralizes or modifies the critic modes. When in healthy adult mode, people can balance needs and responsibilities to engage in reasonable pleasure and productivity activities, such as work, recreation, parenting, sex, self-care, and intellectual and cultural interests (Farrell et al., 2014).

The purpose of this exercise is to help therapists notice, acknowledge, and validate their clients' healthy adult mode behaviors. This helps fortify this mode and emphasize its importance for meeting core needs. For this exercise, the therapist can support and strengthen the client's healthy adult mode by first pointing out and supporting the client's autonomy, such as making decisions, setting limits, and acting to get a need met in a healthy way. After this, the therapist explicitly validates and praises evidence

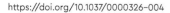

https://doi.org/10.1037/0000326-004

Deliberate Practice in Schema Therapy, by W. T. Behary, J. M. Farrell, A. Vaz, and T. Rousmaniere

of the client's healthy adult mode, as shown in their displays of competence, courage, achievement, limit-setting, self-advocacy, or assertiveness. These interventions are a good opportunity for the person of the therapist to come forth—for example, through the therapist's genuine expression of personal feelings of pride and joy for the client's healthy adult mode.

SKILL CRITERIA FOR EXERCISE 2

1. Support the client's autonomy by pointing out healthy adult mode behaviors (e.g., making decisions, setting limits, acting to get a need met in a healthy way).
2. Validate and praise evidence of the healthy adult mode (e.g., displays of competence, courage, achievement, limit-setting, self-advocacy, assertiveness).

Examples of Supporting and Strengthening the Healthy Adult Mode

Example 1

CLIENT: [*Nervous*] I was tired of the way my husband was treating me. I decided that it was time for me to speak up clearly about what I need from him. I need him to listen when I tell him how I feel and not judge my feelings as right or wrong. I won't accept that anymore.

THERAPIST: So you told him appropriately about a reasonable need. You were clear about your limit. (Criterion 1) I think that's great! Your healthy adult mode is getting stronger. What a good job you did there! (Criterion 2)

Example 2

CLIENT: [*Ashamed*] I was aware that "little me" was triggered when my sister used my embarrassing childhood nickname in front of other people. I felt afraid to tell her that it hurts me, and I felt like running away and hiding. However, I was able to take a breath and told her how I felt and that I don't want her to do that again.

THERAPIST: Wow! You bypassed your fear and spoke from your healthy adult to set a needed limit. (Criterion 1) That is great work. I'm so proud of you. You have a strong and competent healthy adult now to support "little you." (Criterion 2)

Example 3

CLIENT: [*Hesitant*] I want to tell you about what happened yesterday because it's new for me. It may sound small, but for me it was a big deal. I was at dinner with my girlfriend and when we were ordering our meals, she said, "Oh, get the steak not chicken so I can have some of it." I hate it when she tells me what she wants and assumes she can have some of my meal. Usually I give in, but yesterday I simply said, "No, I want the chicken and I intend to eat it all myself." I feel dumb telling you this, but I felt really strong in that moment.

THERAPIST: This does not sound small to me. You spoke up appropriately for what you wanted and have a right to. You did a beautiful job of setting a limit also. (Criterion 1) I am so glad that you felt your strength. Your healthy adult part has a lot of strength, and it is wonderful that you can be an advocate for what you need. Good job! (Criterion 2)

INSTRUCTIONS FOR EXERCISE 2

Step 1: Role-Play and Feedback

- The client says the first beginner client statement. The therapist improvises a response based on the skill criteria.
- The trainer (or, if not available, the client) provides brief feedback based on the skill criteria.
- The client then repeats the same statement, and the therapist again improvises a response. The trainer (or client) again provides brief feedback.

Step 2: Repeat

- Repeat Step 1 for all the statements in the current difficulty level (beginner, intermediate, or advanced).

Step 3: Assess and Adjust Difficulty

- The therapist completes the Deliberate Practice Reaction Form (see Appendix A) and decides whether to make the exercise easier or harder or to repeat the same difficulty level.

Step 4: Repeat for Approximately 15 Minutes

- Repeat Steps 1 to 3 for at least 15 minutes.
- The trainees then switch therapist and client roles and start over.

> **Now it's your turn! Follow Steps 1 and 2 from the instructions.**

Remember: The goal of the role-play is for trainees to practice improvising responses to the client statements in a manner that (a) uses the skill criteria and (b) feels authentic for the trainee. **Example therapist responses for each client statement are provided at the end of this exercise. Trainees should attempt to improvise their own responses before reading the example responses.**

BEGINNER-LEVEL CLIENT STATEMENTS FOR EXERCISE 2
Beginner Client Statement 1
[Hesitant] I think I did a good thing yesterday. My coworker dumped a pile of mail on my desk 15 minutes before the office closed, saying, "I have to leave on time, so I am sure you wouldn't mind dropping these in the mailroom for me." He does things like this all the time, and usually I just do it because "little me" is afraid of him. This time I said "no" quite loudly and started getting ready to leave work.
Beginner Client Statement 2
[Nervous] I was able to tell my wife that I wanted to have sex more often. It is an important part of life, and I don't want us to end up feeling like roommates instead of lovers. She was a bit upset that I was so direct, but it was important to me to let her know how important it is to me. I wasn't critical of her; I just expressed my need.
Beginner Client Statement 3
[Irritated] I decided to finally tell my friend Diana that I am tired of her always being late for our lunch and dinner dates. She was immediately defensive and started making a lot of excuses and even tried to blame me for being so rigid. But I told her it wasn't acceptable. Now, I'm wondering if perhaps I am too rigid? I don't think I am, but I'm not sure. She can be very convincing, just like my mom.
Beginner Client Statement 4
[Upbeat] I was actually able to feel good about myself when I looked in the mirror before walking out the door today. I know it's silly to make a big deal about this, but it felt nice not to be so hard on myself for a change.
Beginner Client Statement 5
[Shy] I visited my aunt last week, and she told me I looked really good. She complimented me on my new haircut. I felt a little uncomfortable at first, like I just wanted to dismiss it as I usually do. But I was able to push myself to thank her and even told her I was very fond of my new haircut too. Wow, am I becoming narcissistic?

 Assess and adjust the difficulty before moving to the next difficulty level (see Step 3 in the exercise instructions).

INTERMEDIATE-LEVEL CLIENT STATEMENTS FOR EXERCISE 2

Intermediate Client Statement 1

[Hesitant] I was feeling kind of needy and sad a few days ago after a really rough period in my relationship. It was as if the little part of me just felt raw from the hard conversations we have been having. I decided that I just needed to stay in bed Saturday and watch children's movies I loved as a kid. At the time I enjoyed it, but now I wonder if it was a healthy thing to do. What do you think?

Intermediate Client Statement 2

[Firm] I have decided to end my friendship with Jane. We have been friends for 10 years, but I realized the last time we went out that she is very critical of me and even mean sometimes. She sounds like my demanding critic mode, and I don't need any reinforcement for that. She puts me down for still being in therapy too. I weighed the pros and cons and decided to end it.

Intermediate Client Statement 3

[Proud] I was really struggling this week with my impulsive child part. All I wanted to do was binge on ice cream. I started out rewarding myself with a scoop of my favorite because I stuck to healthy eating all week. Once I finished that, my little greedy girl wanted more and more. Eventually I said "enough" and threw the rest of the container in the trash. My critic started berating me, but I accessed my internal good parent and told him to shut up.

Intermediate Client Statement 4

[Frustrated] You seem like you are bored with me, and I can feel a part of myself just wanting to become angry and critical of you. I don't like it when I feel like I have to entertain you just like I had to do for my parents my whole life. I thought this was a space where I could just be me.

Intermediate Client Statement 5

[Nervous] I finally spoke up during my evaluation at work. It was a very good evaluation, but once again there was no mention of a promotion, and you know I feel I am way overdue. It was so hard, but suddenly it just came out of me, and I think I said it pretty well because my boss actually smiled and said he would be giving this serious consideration now. Was that a mistake on my part, maybe too pushy and not appreciative?

 Assess and adjust the difficulty before moving to the next difficulty level (see Step 3 in the exercise instructions).

ADVANCED-LEVEL CLIENT STATEMENTS FOR EXERCISE 2
Advanced Client Statement 1
[Firm] I need to raise an issue with you. I have noticed that you often stop our sessions 5 minutes early. Maybe I shouldn't say anything, but I feel that I am not getting all of the allotted time, and it bothers me because I value our session time.
Advanced Client Statement 2
[Gentle] I think you are wrong to tell me that I give in too much to my undisciplined child mode. Is that really what you think? I think it is my little sad child who needs to have fun sometimes and not just work.
Advanced Client Statement 3
[Anxious] What should I do about continuing to go out with Mark? Sometimes I enjoy his company, and feel that he values me, but other times he is bossy and tells me what to do or pushes what he wants sexually. I don't want to lose him, but I don't like the way he treats me sometimes.
Advanced Client Statement 4
[Nervous] I just wanted to get angry and yell when I came home last night to find my wife with that sad look on her face. Once again, I could feel myself being judged and unappreciated by her because I was running late and I forgot to pick up the milk. But then I heard your voice in my head and I took a deep breath and apologized for being late and forgetful. I also promised to go out to get the milk after I had a chance to change my clothes and have a little break. She actually smiled. I couldn't believe it. It felt strange but good. I'm still not sure I will be able to do this again when I am really tired and triggered, though.
Advanced Client Statement 5
[Frustrated] I can't find a way to feel secure since my husband's affair last year. I always feel the urge to check his phone and his laptop, like a spy. I am so tired of this. I finally told him I do not want to be a private investigator for the rest of my life. We need couples therapy if we are going to heal this marriage, or I am not sure I can stay with him. As always, he said I am just paranoid and insecure, but he agreed to go to therapy.

 Assess and adjust the difficulty here (see Step 3 in the exercise instructions). If appropriate, follow the instructions to make the exercise even more challenging (see Appendix A).

Example Therapist Responses: Supporting and Strengthening the Healthy Adult Mode

Remember: Trainees should attempt to improvise their own responses before reading the example responses. **Do not read the following responses verbatim unless you are having trouble coming up with your own responses!**

EXAMPLE RESPONSES TO BEGINNER-LEVEL CLIENT STATEMENTS FOR EXERCISE 2
Example Response to Beginner Client Statement 1
It sounds to me like you set a limit that you have a right to. You were able to connect with the healthy adult part of you even though another part of you felt scared. (Criterion 1) Doing that took courage and deserves applause. Great work! (Criterion 2)
Example Response to Beginner Client Statement 2
You were clear and direct speaking from your healthy adult mode. Sex can be a difficult topic for couples, and you were able to deal with it. (Criterion 1) I admire your ability to express your needs in this important area of life. (Criterion 2)
Example Response to Beginner Client Statement 3
Good for you! Your healthy adult mode was able to advocate for your rights. This is hard, especially with people like Diana and your mom. (Criterion 1) You are not being rigid at all. It's your right to be respected just as you do for her. I am really proud of you. (Criterion 2)
Example Response to Beginner Client Statement 4
Sounds like your healthy adult mode was looking in the mirror, really seeing you—someone who absolutely deserves to feel good about herself. (Criterion 1) That isn't silly at all. It's a big and wonderful step for you, and I couldn't be happier. Thank you for telling me! (Criterion 2)
Example Response to Beginner Client Statement 5
I know the struggle you face whenever someone pays you a compliment. But this time your healthy adult mode was able to accept the message, and that is a big and important step for you. (Criterion 1) This is not at all narcissistic. You actually need to embrace this appreciation for yourself. I am so proud of you for allowing yourself to accept the compliment. (Criterion 2)

EXAMPLE RESPONSES TO INTERMEDIATE-LEVEL CLIENT STATEMENTS FOR EXERCISE 2

Example Response to Intermediate Client Statement 1

I think you took some healthy adult mode actions to soothe the young part of you. It is a good thing to balance stressful events with some soothing restorative time. (Criterion 1). I am happy you did that, and I see it as an accomplishment. You were aware of a need, and you met it in a healthy way. (Criterion 2)

Example Response to Intermediate Client Statement 2

I can imagine that was a difficult decision to make, but also an important one. Your healthy adult mode weighed the pros and cons and came to a balanced decision. (Criterion 1) I think making this decision was an important step for you and one that took courage. Good for you. (Criterion 2)

Example Response to Intermediate Client Statement 3

It sounds like you struggled with a lot of different parts of yourself and, in the end, the healthy adult won out. (Criterion 1) You did a great job of handling your impulsive part and limiting your critic mode. I hope you are pleased with what you accomplished here. (Criterion 2)

Example Response to Intermediate Client Statement 4

Well, that certainly cannot feel good. Thank you for telling me in this way and not just becoming angry and critical. (Criterion 1) I am not at all bored with you, and I'm really glad you shared how you are feeling. I think this is a really important display of your healthy adult part. I'd be happy to talk through this more and pay attention to what I am doing that leads you to feel this way. (Criterion 2)

Example Response to Intermediate Client Statement 5

Well, look at you! Your healthy adult advocate found a welcome place at the table. I know how hard it's been, feeling unworthy of something you've clearly earned the right to have by now. (Criterion 1) What a big step for you. You're really beginning to believe in yourself and that's worthy of a little celebration too. (Criterion 2)

EXAMPLE RESPONSES TO ADVANCED-LEVEL CLIENT STATEMENTS FOR EXERCISE 2

Example Response to Advanced Client Statement 1

You sound strong and definite about this. You also have a right to decide how we use our time together. This is your healthy adult mode. (Criterion 1) I usually allow a few minutes before we end in case something needs to be wrapped up, but we can discuss whether that works for you or not. I am glad you brought this up. (Criterion 2)

Example Response to Advanced Client Statement 2

I am hearing your healthy adult right now. You sound definite about which part of you is involved here, and I accept your assessment. (Criterion 1) Good for you that you have the strength to disagree. I'm glad to hear it. (Criterion 2)

Example Response to Advanced Client Statement 3

You started with a question, but I think you also gave the answer. This is your healthy adult mode. You are clear about what you like and don't like with Mark. (Criterion 1) I'm glad to hear you weighing the pros and cons and realizing that the decision is up to you in the end. (Criterion 2)

Example Response to Advanced Client Statement 4

I know it's hard to imagine being able to be that clear and responsible spokesperson for yourself every time you are upset. That was your healthy adult mode that showed up last night. (Criterion 1) Nobody's perfect, but you are doing beautiful work to address your angry reactions, to be accountable to your loved ones, and also to care for your own needs. I really admire your strength and your progress. (Criterion 2)

Example Response to Advanced Client Statement 5

That is a true victory for you! You expressed your needs, knowing how he was likely to blame you. You are reclaiming your voice and becoming a good advocate for you. This is your healthy adult showing up. (Criterion 1) And now he agreed to couples therapy. No guarantee, but it's a great start to see what's possible in healing the marriage. I know this is important to you, and I am so happy you could stand up for your needs. (Criterion 2)

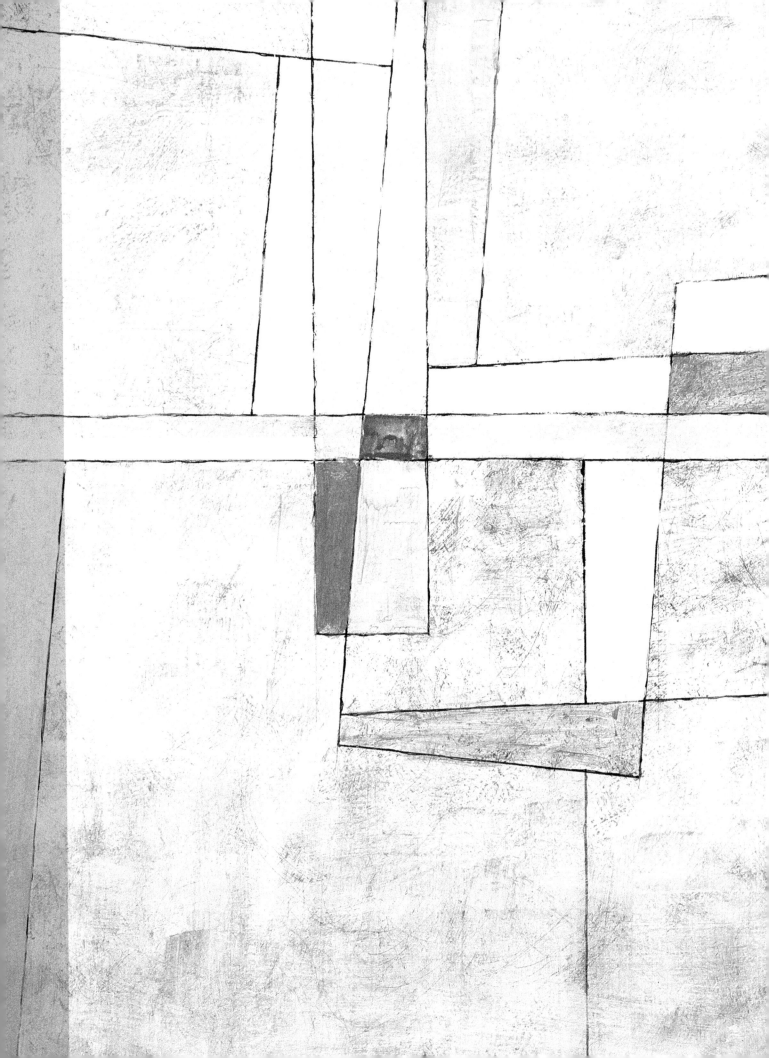

Schema Education: Beginning to Understand Current Problems in Schema Therapy Terms

Preparations for Exercise 3

1. Read the instructions in Chapter 2.

2. Download the Deliberate Practice Reaction Form and Deliberate Practice Diary Form at https://www.apa.org/pubs/books/deliberate-practice-schema-therapy (see the "Clinician and Practitioner Resources" tab; also available in Appendixes A and B, respectively).

Skill Description

Skill Difficulty Level: Beginner

This skill focuses on introducing the client to *early maladaptive schemas* (EMSs). EMSs are core emotional beliefs that, along with biology and temperament, were formed when early emotional needs were not adequately met. Schemas function like personality traits, which contain a person's core beliefs and messages about self, others, and predictions for the future. They may remain dormant for periods of time and become activated under certain conditions that feel reminiscent of painful early life experiences. They can include the activation of distressful feelings, sensations, and biased beliefs, which occur automatically and remain rigidly embedded in the client's sense of what's real. For example, consider a scenario where a client's coworker looks down when she approaches the client's desk, and this triggers the client's sense of rejection and inadequacy (a "defectiveness and abandonment" schema). This leads to feelings of profound hopelessness, anxiety, anger, or loneliness—a long-held reaction arising from early experiences of being significantly deprived and criticized as a little child.

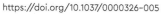

https://doi.org/10.1037/0000326-005
Deliberate Practice in Schema Therapy, by W. T. Behary, J. M. Farrell, A. Vaz, and T. Rousmaniere

In this exercise, the therapist will start the process of making sense of the client's problems in schema therapy terms. The therapist improvises responses following these skill criteria:

1. EMSs often go unchallenged as they operate outside of conscious awareness. The therapist starts by bringing a client's pattern to awareness and naming it a *schema*.

2. The therapist then provides clients with an essential framework for therapy by explaining how schemas originate from early unmet needs. For this exercise, the therapist should practice becoming fluent in providing brief rationales, such as "Schemas develop from the interaction between our biological makeup and emotional needs that were not met in our childhood."

3. The therapist provides the client with education regarding the impact of their schemas on their emotional beliefs and expectations.

You may notice that therapist interventions for this exercise can feel somewhat repetitive across client statements, and this is by design. This exercise provides multiple opportunities to experiment with delivering an essential component of schema education. Future exercises focus on tailoring specific rationales to specific client presentations.

SKILL CRITERIA FOR EXERCISE 3

1. Suggest the presence of a pattern in the client's life, and call this pattern a schema.
2. Explain the origin of schemas in terms of early unmet needs.
3. Educate the client about how schemas are strong emotional beliefs about the self, others, and the world.

Examples of Schema Education: Beginning to Understand Current Problems in Schema Therapy Terms

Example 1

CLIENT: [*Sad*] I have never been able to maintain relationships. I will be lonely and alone forever.

THERAPIST: It sounds like this difficulty in maintaining relationships is a theme in your life, representing what we call a schema. (Criterion 1) Schemas develop from a combination of our biological makeup and the core emotional needs that are not adequately met in our childhood. (Criterion 2) Schemas become intense emotional beliefs that influence the way we see ourselves, the way we relate with others, and even the way we predict our future. (Criterion 3)

Example 2

CLIENT: [*Sad*] No matter how much I try, I can't seem to let anyone care for me. It's like I came into the world expected to be an adult. I had to learn to bury my needs and care for myself.

THERAPIST: It sounds like burying your needs and not letting others care for you is a pattern in your life. We call these patterns a schema. (Criterion 1) Schemas develop in part due to the core emotional needs that were not met in our childhood. (Criterion 2) Schemas are like intense emotional beliefs about yourself and others. They influence your expectations in your current relationships. (Criterion 3)

Example 3

CLIENT: [*Cold*] Well, it's really no surprise that my husband left me. Why would he want to be with someone like me? You will understand better once you really get to know me. Even my mother didn't really like me.

THERAPIST: It sounds like expecting to be disliked or abandoned by others is a theme in your life, or what we call a schema. (Criterion 1) Schemas develop because of our biological makeup and when our core emotional needs are not adequately met in our childhood. (Criterion 2) These schemas create strong emotional beliefs that affect the way we see ourselves, the way we relate with others, and the way we predict our future. (Criterion 3)

INSTRUCTIONS FOR EXERCISE 3

Step 1: Role-Play and Feedback

- The client says the first beginner client statement. The therapist improvises a response based on the skill criteria.
- The trainer (or, if not available, the client) provides brief feedback based on the skill criteria.
- The client then repeats the same statement, and the therapist again improvises a response. The trainer (or client) again provides brief feedback.

Step 2: Repeat

- Repeat Step 1 for all the statements in the current difficulty level (beginner, intermediate, or advanced).

Step 3: Assess and Adjust Difficulty

- The therapist completes the Deliberate Practice Reaction Form (see Appendix A) and decides whether to make the exercise easier or harder or to repeat the same difficulty level.

Step 4: Repeat for Approximately 15 Minutes

- Repeat Steps 1 to 3 for at least 15 minutes.
- The trainees then switch therapist and client roles and start over.

> **Now it's your turn! Follow Steps 1 and 2 from the instructions.**

Remember: The goal of the role-play is for trainees to practice improvising responses to the client statements in a manner that (a) uses the skill criteria and (b) feels authentic for the trainee. **Example therapist responses for each client statement are provided at the end of this exercise. Trainees should attempt to improvise their own responses before reading the example responses.**

BEGINNER-LEVEL CLIENT STATEMENTS FOR EXERCISE 3
Beginner Client Statement 1
[Sad] I have never been able to maintain relationships. I will be lonely and alone forever.
Beginner Client Statement 2
[Hopeless] Anyone I have ever loved has left me or died. There is no use in forming relationships; they never last.
Beginner Client Statement 3
[Irritated] How can you say that I can trust you to be here for me? That has never happened. I know people are unreliable. They can promise they will be there in tough times, but they don't follow through.
Beginner Client Statement 4
[Anxious] I never knew what mood my mother would be in as a child. I learned to brace myself in case it was a day when she wouldn't even talk to me.
Beginner Client Statement 5
[Hopeless] It's just too hard to allow myself to relax and enjoy my new friends. My life has always been about having to pick up and move from one place to another. I know it's just a matter of time before they will change or I will have to move on again.

 Assess and adjust the difficulty before moving to the next difficulty level (see Step 3 in the exercise instructions).

INTERMEDIATE-LEVEL CLIENT STATEMENTS FOR EXERCISE 3
Intermediate Client Statement 1
[Sad] No matter how much I try, I can't seem to let anyone care for me. It's like I came into the world expected to be an adult. I had to learn to bury my needs and care for myself.
Intermediate Client Statement 2
[Hopeless] I feel so empty most of the time. Like I am a hollow person with no warmth or substance. I have nothing to give to a partner and I have never felt cared for or loved. No one was there for me as a kid and now I wouldn't know what to do with expressions of caring. It makes me too uncomfortable.
Intermediate Client Statement 3
[Matter-of-factly] I never had any guidance as a kid, so I learned to make decisions on my own. I realize that this causes me problems in my marriage, but I cannot seem to share the needed information about what I want with my wife. It just doesn't feel natural to me.
Intermediate Client Statement 4
[Cold] I have never found anyone who really understands or accepts me. What is the point of looking for the impossible?
Intermediate Client Statement 5
[Matter-of-factly] I have always had to figure things out for myself. I had to learn to comfort myself when I was scared or worried, from the time I was little. Showing any neediness was not tolerated in my family. In fact, it was treated with annoyance or by just ignoring me.

 Assess and adjust the difficulty before moving to the next difficulty level (see Step 3 in the exercise instructions).

ADVANCED-LEVEL CLIENT STATEMENTS FOR EXERCISE 3
Advanced Client Statement 1
[Cold] Well, it's really no surprise that my husband left me. Why would he want to be with someone like me? You will understand better once you really get to know me. Even my mother didn't really like me.
Advanced Client Statement 2
[Frustrated] I am just a person who has something missing—things I try never work out. My father saw this even when I was a toddler. He never expected much from me, so he focused his attention on my brother.
Advanced Client Statement 3
[Angry] I may as well just face the fact that I am a loser. I have never accomplished as much as my family, and they've always made sure to remind me of that. That old cliche about the "black sheep" fits me perfectly.
Advanced Client Statement 4
[Stressed] I know that you see it too. I am weird. You have probably never tried to work with someone as screwed up as I am. Even my parents gave up on me by the time I was 12.
Advanced Client Statement 5
[Sad] What if I am just someone who doesn't deserve to be loved? I mean, maybe I was just born bad. I certainly was a difficult child who never did anything right and caused a lot of stress, according to my family.

 Assess and adjust the difficulty here (see Step 3 in the exercise instructions). If appropriate, follow the instructions to make the exercise even more challenging (see Appendix A).

Example Therapist Responses: Schema Education: Beginning to Understand Current Problems in Schema Therapy Terms

Remember: Trainees should attempt to improvise their own responses before reading the example responses. **Do not read the following responses verbatim unless you are having trouble coming up with your own responses!**

EXAMPLE RESPONSES TO BEGINNER-LEVEL CLIENT STATEMENTS FOR EXERCISE 3
Example Response to Beginner Client Statement 1
It sounds like you might be describing a pattern or a theme in your life, representing what we call a schema. (Criterion 1) Schemas can develop from a combination of our biological makeup and the core emotional needs that are not adequately met in our childhood. (Criterion 2) Schemas become intense emotional beliefs that influence the way we see ourselves, the way we relate with others, and even the way we predict our future. (Criterion 3)
Example Response to Beginner Client Statement 2
Your experience suggests a pattern that we refer to as a schema. (Criterion 1) It developed from unmet needs in your childhood. (Criterion 2) The schema creates strong beliefs about yourself and your future, including your belief that no relationship will last. (Criterion 3)
Example Response to Beginner Client Statement 3
Your reaction is part of a pattern we call a schema. (Criterion 1) It developed in part because of your childhood experiences and early unmet needs. (Criterion 2) This schema leads to strong beliefs and expectations in your current life, like this belief that everyone will leave you. (Criterion 3)
Example Response to Beginner Client Statement 4
This anxiety reflects the presence of a schema. (Criterion 1) It developed because your normal childhood needs were not met growing up. (Criterion 2) This schema leads to your current beliefs about yourself and others. (Criterion 3)
Example Response to Beginner Client Statement 5
This pattern of difficulty feeling secure in relationships suggests the presence of a schema. (Criterion 1) This schema was probably formed in your childhood because of your early unmet needs. (Criterion 2) Schemas create strong emotional beliefs about yourself, others, and your expectations for the future. (Criterion 3)

EXAMPLE RESPONSES TO INTERMEDIATE-LEVEL CLIENT STATEMENTS FOR EXERCISE 3

Example Response to Intermediate Client Statement 1

It sounds like a pattern in your life, representing what we call a schema. (Criterion 1) Schemas develop from the interaction between our biological makeup and the core emotional needs that were not met in our childhood. (Criterion 2) Schemas are like intense emotional beliefs about yourself and others. They influence your expectations in your current relationships. (Criterion 3)

Example Response to Intermediate Client Statement 2

These feelings and your difficulty accepting caring from others indicate a pattern that we call a schema. (Criterion 1) It developed because your normal childhood need for care, nurture, and love was not met. (Criterion 2) From that unmet need, you developed strong emotional beliefs—which are part of what we call a schema—about yourself and others that keep you in this empty state. (Criterion 3)

Example Response to Intermediate Client Statement 3

This difficulty comes from what we call a schema. (Criterion 1) Your normal needs for guidance were not met in childhood, (Criterion 2) so you developed a schema, which includes strong beliefs about how relationships work and how you operate in them. (Criterion 3)

Example Response to Intermediate Client Statement 4

This pattern you're describing is a schema operating. (Criterion 1) Schemas are formed from not having your normal needs for understanding and acceptance met as a child. (Criterion 2) This schema leads to your current beliefs about yourself and others, such as this belief that you cannot get these things from other people. (Criterion 3)

Example Response to Intermediate Client Statement 5

This is an example of what we refer to as a schema. (Criterion 1) Your childhood needs for emotional support and comfort were not met. (Criterion 2) These experiences created a schema, a strong emotional belief that no one will be there for you. (Criterion 3)

EXAMPLE RESPONSES TO ADVANCED-LEVEL CLIENT STATEMENTS FOR EXERCISE 3

Example Response to Advanced Client Statement 1

Seeing yourself as unlikable seems like a pattern or a theme in your life—what we call a schema. (Criterion 1) Schemas are formed from our biological makeup and core emotional needs that are not adequately met in our childhood. (Criterion 2) This schema is a strong emotional belief that causes you to see yourself as unlikable and think that other people see you that way as well. (Criterion 3)

Example Response to Advanced Client Statement 2

This sounds like a pattern of viewing yourself negatively. It's an example of what we call a schema. (Criterion 1) It developed because your normal childhood needs were not met. (Criterion 2) This led to some strong beliefs about yourself, such as the belief that you are unworthy. (Criterion 3)

Example Response to Advanced Client Statement 3

What you're describing, this pattern or theme in your life, is what we call a schema. (Criterion 1) Schemas develop when childhood needs are not met, like your not receiving positive feedback and nurturance. (Criterion 2) Schemas are intense emotional beliefs about oneself and the world. For example, your schemas influence you to accept this negative view of yourself as truth. (Criterion 3)

Example Response to Advanced Client Statement 4

This sounds like a pattern of seeing yourself as flawed and assuming that is what others see. We call this a schema. (Criterion 1) It developed because your normal need for love and to be valued was not met in childhood. (Criterion 2) These unmet needs led to you developing this belief about yourself as "weird." (Criterion 3)

Example Response to Advanced Client Statement 5

This painful idea, that you are innately bad and unlovable, is an example of a schema. (Criterion 1) This schema developed because your childhood needs for love and support were not met. (Criterion 2) It led you to have biased beliefs that your struggles as a child were your fault and that you were flawed. (Criterion 3)

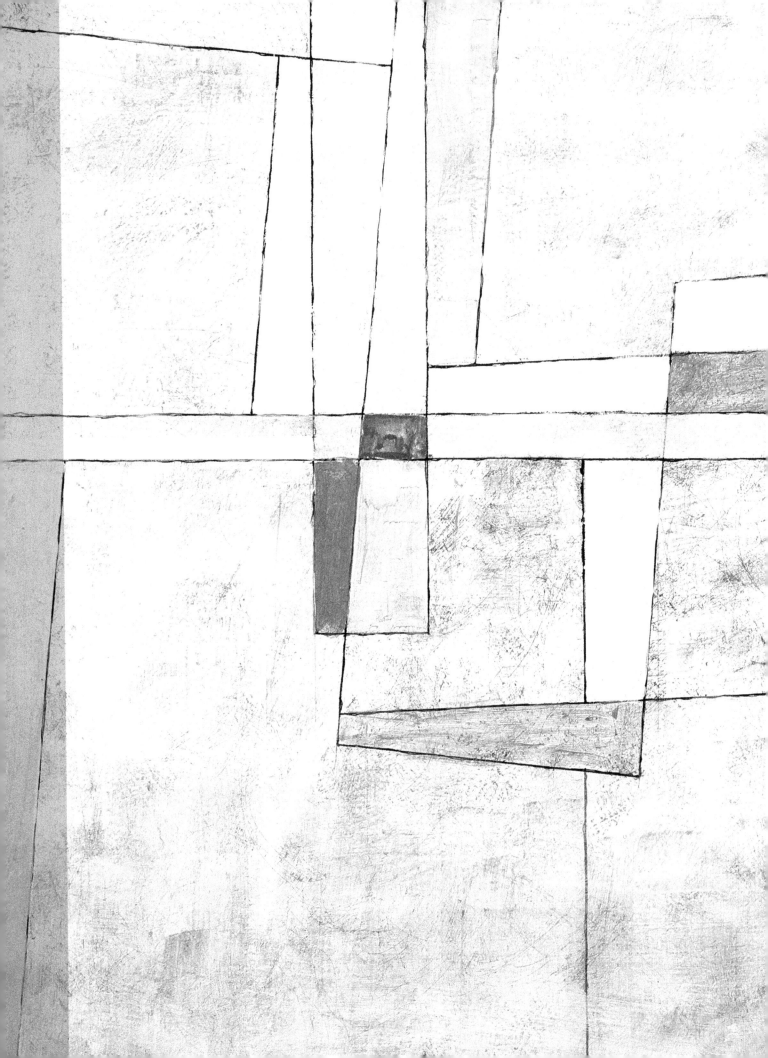

Linking Unmet Needs, Schema, and Presenting Problem

Preparations for Exercise 4

1. Read the instructions in Chapter 2.

2. Download the Deliberate Practice Reaction Form and Deliberate Practice Diary Form at https://www.apa.org/pubs/books/deliberate-practice-schema-therapy (see the "Clinician and Practitioner Resources" tab; also available in Appendixes A and B, respectively).

Skill Description

Skill Difficulty Level: Beginner

This skill focuses on linking the client's unmet childhood needs and the related schema belief to the client's presenting problem. This is the beginning of translating the client's view of their problem into the concepts of schema therapy. Establishing this schema language early in therapy provides clients with a framework to help make sense of their problems, thereby facilitating a positive therapeutic alliance.

In this exercise, the therapist explains the role of the client's early unmet needs in the development of a schema. Having done this, the therapist then suggests a link between this schema with possible current problems in the client's life.

Each difficulty level of client statements in this exercise reflects one of three schemas:

- abandonment/instability schema (beginner client statements)
- emotional deprivation schema (intermediate client statements)
- defectiveness/shame schema (advanced client statements)

https://doi.org/10.1037/0000326-006

Deliberate Practice in Schema Therapy, by W. T. Behary, J. M. Farrell, A. Vaz, and T. Rousmaniere

Understanding the core components of each schema helps therapists link the client's unmet needs with their current presenting problems, so we briefly define the schemas next. (For more information on core ST concepts, see Appendix C of this book.)

Abandonment/Instability Schema

Definition

This schema involves the feeling that significant others will not be able to continue providing emotional support, connection, strength, or practical protection because they are emotionally unstable and unpredictable, unreliable, or erratically present; because they will die imminently; or because they will abandon you in favor of someone better.

Related Unmet Need

Development of this schema is often connected with childhood experiences or perceptions that the people needed for support and connection are unstable, unpredictable, or unreliable.

Emotional Deprivation Schema

Definition

This schema involves the "expectation that one's desire for emotional support will not be adequately met by others" (Young et al., 2003, p. 14).

Related Unmet Need

Development of this schema is connected to three major forms of deprivation:

- deprivation of nurturance: absence of attention, affection, warmth, or companionship
- deprivation of empathy: absence of understanding, listening, self-disclosure, or mutual sharing of feelings from others
- deprivation of protection: absence of strength, direction, or guidance from others

Defectiveness/Shame Schema

Definition

This schema entails "feeling that one is defective, bad, unwanted, inferior, or invalid in important respects or that one would be unlovable to significant others if exposed" (Young et al., 2003, p. 15). This schema "may involve hypersensitivity to criticism, rejection, and blame; self-consciousness, comparisons, and insecurity around others; or a sense of shame regarding one's perceived flaws" (Young et al., 2003, p. 15).

Related Unmet Need

This schema is associated with the unmet need to be accepted, praised, and made to feel that they are loveable.

SKILL CRITERIA FOR EXERCISE 4

1. Validate the importance of needs that were unmet in the client's childhood experience.
2. Suggest a link between the client's early unmet needs and the development of a schema.
3. Suggest a link between the client's schema and possible problems in their adult life.

Examples of Linking Unmet Needs, Schema, and Presenting Problem

Example 1: Abandonment/Instability Schema

CLIENT: [*Sad*] I have felt lonely all my life. My family moved a lot because of my dad's job. Nothing ever felt stable. It was hard to form friendships and I often felt left out. To be honest, I feel I'll be alone forever.

THERAPIST: All children have a need for stability—having people to count on and connect with in a predictable and consistent way. With all of the moves you experienced, this need was not adequately met for you. (Criterion 1) This probably led to the development of an abandonment/instability schema. (Criterion 2) When this schema is triggered now or when you are feeling lonely, it leaves you believing that you will be alone forever. (Criterion 3)

Example 2: Emotional Deprivation Schema

CLIENT: [*Sad*] It's like I came into the world expected to be an adult. I never got any nurturing, attention, guidance, or affection. My mom was very depressed when I was young, and my dad was always focused on his work. I was left to figure out how to care for myself. Nowadays, I can't seem to let anyone care for me. I am just not used to it.

THERAPIST: All children need nurturing, attention, guidance, and affection. These seem to have been missing in your childhood. (Criterion 1) When these needs are unmet, a child can form what we call an emotional deprivation schema. (Criterion 2) You learned so young that you couldn't count on the adults in your life to meet your needs, and now when that schema is activated, it's hard for you to accept that others might really care about you. (Criterion 3)

Example 3: Defectiveness/Shame Schema

CLIENT: [*Frustrated*] My father never expected much from me, so he focused his attention on my brother. He would always make jokes about me when I would get upset. He told me I was weak and that I wasn't as smart as my older brother. He basically made me feel like I was a loser. I think he may have been right. Things I try will never work out.

THERAPIST: All children have the need to be accepted, praised, and made to feel that they are loveable. Unfortunately, it seems you didn't get these important needs met early on. (Criterion 1) When that happens, children can develop a schema called defectiveness/shame. (Criterion 2) When this schema is activated today, it causes intense painful emotions with the underlying belief that you are not good enough and not worthy of love or attention. Based on these experiences and this schema, no wonder you sometimes feel like things you try will never work out. (Criterion 3)

INSTRUCTIONS FOR EXERCISE 4

Step 1: Role-Play and Feedback

- The client says the first beginner client statement. The therapist improvises a response based on the skill criteria.
- The trainer (or, if not available, the client) provides brief feedback based on the skill criteria.
- The client then repeats the same statement, and the therapist again improvises a response. The trainer (or client) again provides brief feedback.

Step 2: Repeat

- Repeat Step 1 for all the statements in the current difficulty level (beginner, intermediate, or advanced).

Step 3: Assess and Adjust Difficulty

- The therapist completes the Deliberate Practice Reaction Form (see Appendix A) and decides whether to make the exercise easier or harder or to repeat the same difficulty level.

Step 4: Repeat for Approximately 15 Minutes

- Repeat Steps 1 to 3 for at least 15 minutes.
- The trainees then switch therapist/client roles and start over.

> **Now it's your turn! Follow Steps 1 and 2 from the instructions.**

Remember: The goal of the role-play is for trainees to practice improvising responses to the client statements in a manner that (a) uses the skill criteria and (b) feels authentic for the trainee. **Example therapist responses for each client statement are provided at the end of this exercise. Trainees should attempt to improvise their own responses before reading the example responses.**

BEGINNER-LEVEL CLIENT STATEMENTS FOR EXERCISE 4: ABANDONMENT/INSTABILITY SCHEMA
Beginner Client Statement 1
[Sad] I have felt lonely all my life. My family moved a lot because of my dad's job. Nothing ever felt stable. It was hard to form friendships, and I often felt left out. To be honest, I feel like I'll be alone forever.
Beginner Client Statement 2
[Hopeless] Anyone I have ever loved has left me or died. There is no use in forming relationships.
Beginner Client Statement 3
[Irritated] I know people are unreliable. My dad promised to always be there for me, and then he disappeared from my life when I was still a kid. People promise they will be there in tough times, but they don't follow through.
Beginner Client Statement 4
[Anxious] I never knew what mood my mother would be in as a child. I learned to brace myself in case it was a day when she wouldn't even talk to me. To this day, I still worry about people being unpredictable. Honestly, I think that's what makes me so nervous about coming in to see you.
Beginner Client Statement 5
[Hopeless] It's just too hard to allow myself to relax and enjoy my new friends. My life has always been about having to pick up and move from one place to another. I know it's just a matter of time before they will change, or I will have to move on again.

 Assess and adjust the difficulty before moving to the next difficulty level (see Step 3 in the exercise instructions).

INTERMEDIATE-LEVEL CLIENT STATEMENTS FOR EXERCISE 4: EMOTIONAL DEPRIVATION SCHEMA

Intermediate Client Statement 1

[Sad] It's like I came into the world expected to be an adult. I never got any attention or guidance. My mom was very depressed when I was young, and my dad was always focused on his work. I was left to figure out how to care for myself. Nowadays, I can't seem to let anyone care for me. I am just not used to it.

Intermediate Client Statement 2

[Hopeless] I have never found anyone who really understands or accepts me. My family sure didn't. What is the point of looking for the impossible?

Intermediate Client Statement 3

[Matter-of-factly] I never had any guidance as a kid, so I learned to make decisions on my own. I realize that this causes problems in my marriage, but I can't seem to share what I need with my wife. It just doesn't feel natural to me.

Intermediate Client Statement 4

[Sad] I have nothing to give to a partner and I have never felt cared for or loved. No one was there for me as a kid, and now I wouldn't know what to do with expressions of caring. It makes me too uncomfortable.

> 🛑 **Assess and adjust the difficulty before moving to the next difficulty level (see Step 3 in the exercise instructions).**

ADVANCED-LEVEL CLIENT STATEMENTS FOR EXERCISE 4: DEFECTIVENESS/SHAME SCHEMA
Advanced Client Statement 1
[Matter-of-factly] I have always had to figure things out for myself. I had to learn to comfort myself when I was scared or worried, from the time I was little. Showing any neediness was not tolerated in my family; in fact, it was treated with annoyance or by just ignoring me.
Advanced Client Statement 2
[Frustrated] My father never expected much from me, so he focused his attention on my brother. He would always make jokes about me when I would get upset, told me I was weak, and that I wasn't as smart as my older brother. He basically made me feel like I was a loser. I think he may have been right. Things I try will never work out.
Advanced Client Statement 3
[Depressed] Well, it's really no surprise that my husband left me. Why would he want to be with someone like me? You will understand better once you really get to know me. Even my mother didn't really like me.
Advanced Client Statement 4
[Angry] I may as well just face the fact that I am a loser. I've never accomplished as much as my family, and they've always made sure to remind me of that. That old cliché about the black sheep fits me perfectly.
Advanced Client Statement 5
[Stressed] I'm weird. I know that you see it too. You've probably never tried to work with someone as screwed up as I am. Even my parents gave up on me by the time I was 12.
Advanced Client Statement 6
[Sad] What if I am just someone who doesn't deserve to be loved? I mean, maybe I was just born bad. I certainly was a difficult child who never did anything right, according to my family.

 Assess and adjust the difficulty here (see Step 3 in the exercise instructions). If appropriate, follow the instructions to make the exercise even more challenging (see Appendix A).

Example Therapist Responses: Linking Unmet Needs, Schema, and Presenting Problem

Remember: Trainees should attempt to improvise their own responses before reading the example responses. **Do not read the following responses verbatim unless you are having trouble coming up with your own responses!**

EXAMPLE RESPONSES TO BEGINNER-LEVEL CLIENT STATEMENTS FOR EXERCISE 4: ABANDONMENT/INSTABILITY SCHEMA
Example Response to Beginner Client Statement 1
All children have a need for stability—having people to count on and connect with in a predictable and consistent way. With all the moves you experienced, this need was not adequately met for you. (Criterion 1) This probably led to the development of an abandonment/instability schema. (Criterion 2) When this schema is triggered now or when you are feeling lonely, it leaves you believing that you will be alone forever. (Criterion 3)
Example Response to Beginner Client Statement 2
Every child needs to know that there is someone they can count on in a predictable and stable way, someone who will not go away. (Criterion 1) Given the losses you've suffered, this need was not met, leading to the development of an abandonment/instability schema. (Criterion 2) The thought of forming new relationships today triggers this schema, and you feel it's useless. (Criterion 3)
Example Response to Beginner Client Statement 3
Every child needs to feel that there is someone who will be there for them, someone they can count on, someone who will not go away. (Criterion 1) In your early life, your dad didn't keep his promises, leading you to develop an abandonment/instability schema. (Criterion 2) It's hard to imagine that anyone can really be trusted to be there for you when this schema gets triggered. (Criterion 3)
Example Response to Beginner Client Statement 4
Every child needs their parent to be stable, to be present and attuned. (Criterion 1) Given your mother's unpredictable moods, you developed an abandonment/instability schema. (Criterion 2) The triggering of this schema leads you to feel as if even I might not be reliable, that I might turn away from you. (Criterion 3)
Example Response to Beginner Client Statement 5
All children have a need for stability—having people to count on and connect with consistently. (Criterion 1) Given all the moves and losses you experienced as a child, this need was not adequately met for you, leading to the abandonment/instability schema. (Criterion 2) When this schema is triggered now, you believe that your relationships will inevitably end. (Criterion 3)

EXAMPLE RESPONSES TO INTERMEDIATE-LEVEL CLIENT STATEMENTS FOR EXERCISE 4: EMOTIONAL DEPRIVATION SCHEMA

Example Response to Intermediate Client Statement 1

All children need nurturing, attention, guidance, and affection. These seem to have been missing in your childhood. (Criterion 1) When these needs are unmet, a child can form what we call an emotional deprivation schema. (Criterion 2) You learned so young that you couldn't count on the adults in your life to meet your needs, and now when that schema is activated, it's hard for you to accept that others might really care about you. (Criterion 3)

Example Response to Intermediate Client Statement 2

All children need to feel understood and accepted. (Criterion 1) Not getting this need met as a child leads to the development of an emotional deprivation schema. (Criterion 2) When this schema is triggered now, you feel that it's not worth trying to connect with anyone because you believe they will also not be able to see you or accept you. (Criterion 3)

Example Response to Intermediate Client Statement 3

Every child needs to have the guidance and support of their caregivers. This prepares a child to be able to connect and to be autonomous. (Criterion 1) Not having this guidance in your early life led you to develop an emotional deprivation schema. (Criterion 2) When triggered in your marriage, it causes you to struggle with asking for what you need. (Criterion 3)

Example Response to Intermediate Client Statement 4

Every child needs to feel seen, loved, and cared for, to be treasured for just being the precious little one that they are. (Criterion 1) This need was not adequately met for you, leading to what we call an emotional deprivation schema—an intense emotional belief that no one can be counted on for love and caring. (Criterion 2) Now, when someone shows caring when you need it, the schema gets triggered, leaving you confused and uncomfortable. (Criterion 3)

EXAMPLE RESPONSES TO ADVANCED-LEVEL CLIENT STATEMENTS FOR EXERCISE 4: DEFECTIVENESS/SHAME SCHEMA
Example Response to Advanced Client Statement 1
All children need to know that their feelings matter, to be accepted and loved when they are happy, scared, angry, or sad. (Criterion 1) You were made to feel as if you were doing something wrong when you were scared or worried, leading to the development of a defectiveness/shame schema. (Criterion 2) Given your early experiences, when this schema is activated, you may feel that you can't express your feelings or allow someone else to comfort you. (Criterion 3)
Example Response to Advanced Client Statement 2
All children have the need to be accepted, praised, and made to feel that they are loveable. Unfortunately, it seems you didn't get these important needs met early on. (Criterion 1) When that happens, children can develop a schema called defectiveness/shame. (Criterion 2) When this schema is activated today, it causes intense painful emotions with the underlying belief that you are not good enough, and not worthy of love or attention. Given these experiences and this schema, no wonder you sometimes feel like things you try will never work out. (Criterion 3)
Example Response to Advanced Client Statement 3
All children need to know that they are loveable. (Criterion 1) Given your experiences with your mother, this need was not met, probably leading to a defectiveness/shame schema. (Criterion 2) Now, the schema gets triggered, and you take the blame for your husband's decision, just as you were taught to believe when you were a child. (Criterion 3)
Example Response to Advanced Client Statement 4
Every child needs to feel that they are loveable and acceptable without meeting any conditions, without having to compete or prove themselves. (Criterion 1) Being treated like you were inferior to your family members led to the development of a defectiveness/shame schema. (Criterion 2) When this schema is activated today, you may struggle with believing that you are "a loser" and not good enough. (Criterion 3)
Example Response to Advanced Client Statement 5
All children need to feel love and acceptance from their caregivers. (Criterion 1) You were made to feel as if you were unacceptable at an early age, leading to a schema called defectiveness/shame. (Criterion 2) When this schema is triggered, even in your interactions with me, it leaves you feeling as if you are inadequate and unacceptable. (Criterion 3)
Example Response to Advanced Client Statement 6
All children are born innocent and vulnerable, with the need and the right to be loved and cared for. No child is born bad. (Criterion 1) Given this unmet need in your early life, you developed a schema that we call defectiveness/shame. (Criterion 2) It has led to a lifetime of feeling that you are not worthy of being loved, like you've done something wrong. (Criterion 3)

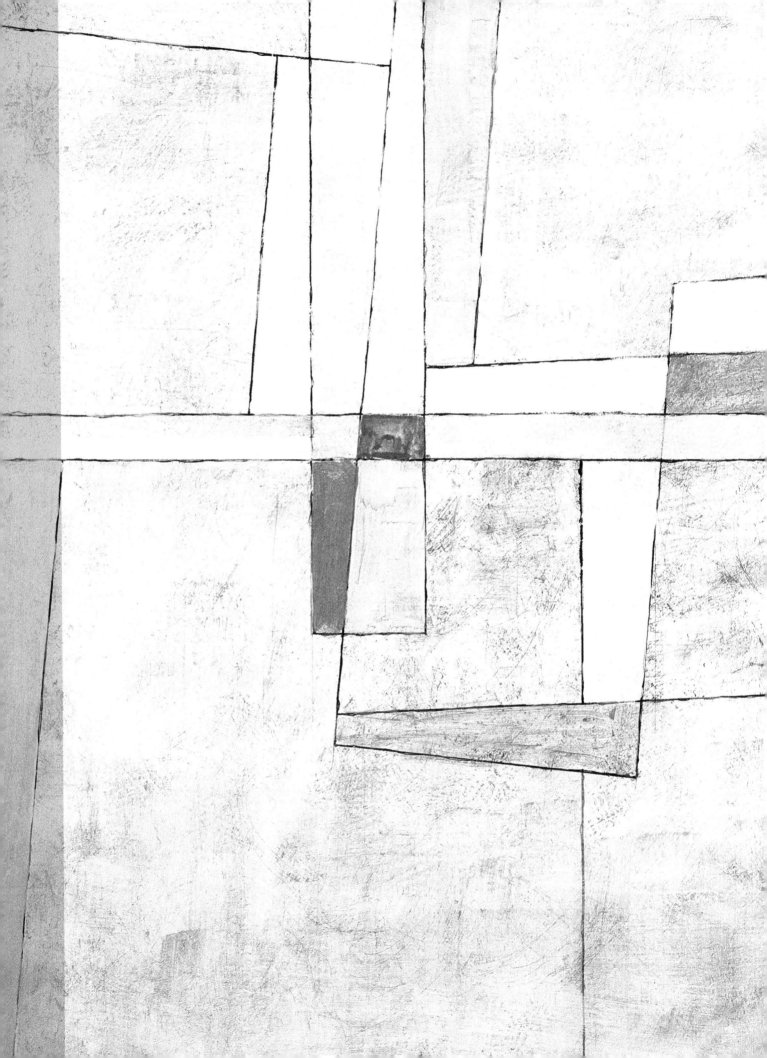

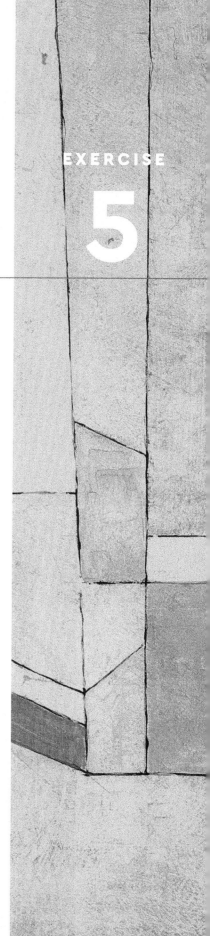

Education About Maladaptive Schema Modes

Preparations for Exercise 5

1. Read the instructions in Chapter 2.

2. Download the Deliberate Practice Reaction Form and Deliberate Practice Diary Form at https://www.apa.org/pubs/books/deliberate-practice-schema-therapy (see the "Clinician and Practitioner Resources" tab; also available in Appendixes A and B, respectively).

Skill Description

Skill Difficulty Level: Intermediate

This skill focuses on introducing the client to the concept of *schema modes*. Referred to simply as *modes*, they are defined as the current emotional, cognitive, behavioral, and neurobiological state that a person experiences. In other words, modes are transient states, in contrast to schemas, which are more akin to stable traits. Modes can be maladaptive or healthy and adaptive. Maladaptive modes are aspects of the self that are not entirely integrated and occur most frequently when multiple maladaptive schemas are activated. Maladaptive modes are characterized by intense distressing or painful emotions, harsh and/or critical thoughts and messages, or problematic or extreme behavior. It is important for the therapist to point out the triggering or rapid shift into maladaptive modes when they occur, so that the client can become aware of them. This awareness is an important early step toward healthy change in the schema therapy model.

For this exercise, the therapist improvises a response to each client statement following these skill criteria:

1. Start your interventions by bringing awareness to the activation of a maladaptive schema mode. A triggered mode is often seen through the client's emotional intensity, disconnection, or extreme critical thoughts.

https://doi.org/10.1037/0000326-007
Deliberate Practice in Schema Therapy, by W. T. Behary, J. M. Farrell, A. Vaz, and T. Rousmaniere

2. Educate clients about the basics of scheme modes. This, along with educating clients on schemas themselves (see Exercises 2 and 3 in this book), provides clients with a rationale for their intense reactions and experiences that may have otherwise felt incomprehensible to them.

SKILL CRITERIA FOR EXERCISE 5

1. Point out the client's behaviors that suggest a maladaptive mode has been triggered.
2. Explain the basic definition of schema modes in terms of parts of self or transient states that are triggered when schemas are activated.

Examples of Education About Maladaptive Schema Modes

Example 1

CLIENT: [*Hopeless*] I waited all weekend for my boyfriend to call me. His rejection is so humiliating. The more I talk about it, the more I just feel so worthless.

THERAPIST: It sounds like you are feeling this intense sense of hopelessness right now. (Criterion 1) This is an example of what we refer to as a mode. Modes are emotional, cognitive, or behavioral states that are triggered when our schemas are activated. (Criterion 2)

Example 2

CLIENT: [*Self-critical*] I'm just not prepared for this interview, and I really need this job. What was I thinking? I will make a fool of myself. What's wrong with me?

THERAPIST: There's that part of you harshly criticizing you in a nonhelpful way. (Criterion 1) This part is what we call a schema mode. A mode is part of you that developed in childhood, when negative messages about us are formed. (Criterion 2)

Example 3

CLIENT: [*Angry*] I feel very angry right now when I think about how little safety I had as a child. It was criminal the way I was treated. It was so unfair! My parents should be in jail.

THERAPIST: It sounds like you are feeling the intense anger you couldn't express as a child. (Criterion 1) This is what we refer to as a schema mode, and it is triggered in response to schemas activated by memories of your childhood needs not being met. (Criterion 2)

INSTRUCTIONS FOR EXERCISE 5
Step 1: Role-Play and Feedback
• The client says the first beginner client statement. The therapist improvises a response based on the skill criteria.
• The trainer (or, if not available, the client) provides brief feedback based on the skill criteria.
• The client then repeats the same statement, and the therapist again improvises a response. The trainer (or client) again provides brief feedback.
Step 2: Repeat
• Repeat Step 1 for all the statements in the current difficulty level (beginner, intermediate, or advanced).
Step 3: Assess and Adjust Difficulty
• The therapist completes the Deliberate Practice Reaction Form (see Appendix A) and decides whether to make the exercise easier or harder or to repeat the same difficulty level.
Step 4: Repeat for Approximately 15 Minutes
• Repeat Steps 1 to 3 for at least 15 minutes.
• The trainees then switch therapist and client roles and start over.

> **Now it's your turn! Follow Steps 1 and 2 from the instructions.**

Remember: The goal of the role-play is for trainees to practice improvising responses to the client statements in a manner that (a) uses the skill criteria and (b) feels authentic for the trainee. **Example therapist responses for each client statement are provided at the end of this exercise. Trainees should attempt to improvise their own responses before reading the example responses.**

BEGINNER-LEVEL CLIENT STATEMENTS FOR EXERCISE 5
Beginner Client Statement 1
[Hopeless] I waited all weekend for my boyfriend to call me. His rejection is so humiliating. The more I talk about it, the more I just feel so worthless.
Beginner Client Statement 2
[Sad] I never felt loved as a child or that I mattered to anyone. I have such a horrible sinking feeling just remembering it.
Beginner Client Statement 3
[Angry] I feel very angry right now when I think about how little safety I had as a child. It was criminal the way I was treated. It was so unfair! My parents should be in jail.
Beginner Client Statement 4
[Angry] Once again, no one invited me to lunch today. My coworkers make their lunch plans and overlook me like I'm invisible. You know what? Who needs them! They are all boring and not very interesting anyway. They are just jealous of me.
Beginner Client Statement 5
[Hopeless] I don't know why I expected the date to go well. I should just accept that I am a loser who no one wants to be around. Even my mother didn't particularly like me and said I was a disappointment.

> **Assess and adjust the difficulty before moving to the next difficulty level (see Step 3 in the exercise instructions).**

INTERMEDIATE-LEVEL CLIENT STATEMENTS FOR EXERCISE 5
Intermediate Client Statement 1
[Self-critical] I'm just not prepared for this job interview, and I really need this job. What was I thinking? I will make a fool of myself. What's wrong with me?
Intermediate Client Statement 2
[Self-disparaging] I have been feeling upset since the divorce, but I know I am making a big deal of it and acting like a whiner. I should just be able to get on with my life.
Intermediate Client Statement 3
[Upset] It's just so hard to believe that my best friend of 30 years is really moving so far away next month. I cannot imagine how I will get on with my life without her steady support. It's like my dad leaving us all those years ago.
Intermediate Client Statement 4
[Angry] I told you that I don't feel things; I'm not sure why you keep asking about my feelings. This emotional stuff is just not for me. I have a very busy life.
Intermediate Client Statement 5
[Calm] I am not really sure why I'm here. I can't really come up with any goals for myself. [Suddenly self-critical] I am such a waste of a human. My dad was right, I'm such a waste.

 Assess and adjust the difficulty before moving to the next difficulty level (see Step 3 in the exercise instructions).

ADVANCED-LEVEL CLIENT STATEMENTS FOR EXERCISE 5

Advanced Client Statement 1

[Angry] I can't believe you are taking vacation time this month when I am dealing with so much stress and I am so alone. You say you care about me, but you are just like everyone else. I hate you.

Advanced Client Statement 2

[Positive] I get a lot out of our sessions. I feel safe here. [Suddenly anxious] But maybe I'm becoming too dependent on you. Why don't we change our sessions to once a month?

Advanced Client Statement 3

[Fearful] I am so afraid that I will also drive you away, just like everyone else in my life. [Suddenly self-critical] You must be so fed up with me. I know I have made some progress, but I don't try hard enough. All I do is whine about my life.

Advanced Client Statement 4

[Anxious] I had a terrible nightmare last night that the older cousin who sexually abused me was at the door of my house. All day I have felt scared and jumpy. [Suddenly becomes flat] Oh, I'm just being stupid. That happened years ago. I have no reason to feel anything about it. No big deal.

Advanced Client Statement 5

[Guilty] I would love to sleep a little later on Saturdays and enjoy some time with my husband, but my mom gets so depressed when I don't call her early in the morning. She really needs me, and always has. I feel so guilty just talking about it now.

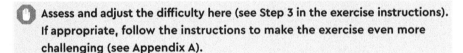 **Assess and adjust the difficulty here (see Step 3 in the exercise instructions). If appropriate, follow the instructions to make the exercise even more challenging (see Appendix A).**

Example Therapist Responses: Education About Maladaptive Schema Modes

Remember: Trainees should attempt to improvise their own responses before reading the example responses. **Do not read the following responses verbatim unless you are having trouble coming up with your own responses!**

EXAMPLE RESPONSES TO BEGINNER-LEVEL CLIENT STATEMENTS FOR EXERCISE 5
Example Response to Beginner Client Statement 1
It sounds like you are feeling an intense sense of hopelessness. (Criterion 1) This state is an example of what we refer to as a mode. Modes are emotional, cognitive, or behavioral states that are triggered when our schemas are activated. (Criterion 2).
Example Response to Beginner Client Statement 2
So you're really feeling these painful emotions right now, as you remember your childhood. (Criterion 1) This is an example of what we refer to as a mode being triggered. (Criterion 2)
Example Response to Beginner Client Statement 3
It sounds like you are feeling the intense anger, which you couldn't express as a child. (Criterion 1) This is what we refer to as a schema mode. This is a state that gets activated in response to memories of your childhood needs not being met. (Criterion 2)
Example Response to Beginner Client Statement 4
I can really hear your anger coming up as you describe this. (Criterion 1) This is what we call a schema mode. Modes are triggered when schemas are activated in response to a triggering event. (Criterion 2)
Example Response to Beginner Client Statement 5
That sounds really harsh and too extreme a judgment. (Criterion 1) I think a mode has been triggered—the part of you that comes up when you feel less than perfect and a schema is activated. (Criterion 2)

EXAMPLE RESPONSES TO INTERMEDIATE-LEVEL CLIENT STATEMENTS FOR EXERCISE 5
Example Response to Intermediate Client Statement 1
You just shifted to a part of you that is harshly critical in a nonhelpful way. (Criterion 1) This part is what we call a schema mode. A mode is a part of us that developed in childhood when negative messages about us are formed. (Criterion 2)
Example Response to Intermediate Client Statement 2
I hear a part of yourself that judges you harshly. (Criterion 1) This part is what we call a schema mode. It formed from childhood experiences where needs were not met. (Criterion 2)
Example Response to Intermediate Client Statement 3
I notice that you seem upset as you describe this to me and are reminded of an earlier loss. (Criterion 1) I think that you switched to another part of yourself, a schema mode, which formed when you were young and struggling with loss. (Criterion 2)
Example Response to Intermediate Client Statement 4
I notice that you became angry. (Criterion 1) This angry side could be a schema mode, a part of you that shows up to keep you from exposing any vulnerability. This might be something you learned in your early childhood as a way of dealing with emotions. (Criterion 2)
Example Response to Intermediate Client Statement 5
It sounds like you are in a very self-critical state. (Criterion 1) This might be a schema mode, something you learned to do when you were young. (Criterion 2)

EXAMPLE RESPONSES TO ADVANCED-LEVEL CLIENT STATEMENTS FOR EXERCISE 5
Example Response to Advanced Client Statement 1
I can see how upset and alone you feel thinking about my absence. (Criterion 1) This reaction is a schema mode, which gets triggered when you sense a possible loss in an important relationship. It is the part of you that reacts to your schemas being activated. (Criterion 2)
Example Response to Advanced Client Statement 2
You seem to have fears about closeness. (Criterion 1) I think that you flipped to what we call a schema mode. This mode is a part of you that fears and avoids closeness and is triggered when schemas are activated. (Criterion 2)
Example Response to Advanced Client Statement 3
I hear you being harshly judgmental and critical of yourself. (Criterion 1) I think that the part of you that is triggered when schemas related to self-criticism are activated. We refer to this reaction as a schema mode. (Criterion 2)
Example Response to Advanced Client Statement 4
It seems like you are criticizing yourself for having feelings. (Criterion 1) That harsh part of you is a schema mode. It was triggered when some of your schemas related to having feelings were activated. (Criterion 2)
Example Response to Advanced Client Statement 5
Sounds like a reasonable wish, to want to have a little time for yourself, but you have a lot of guilt about it. (Criterion 1) This could be a schema mode that was developed in your early relationship with your mom. A mode is like a part of you that gets triggered whenever your schemas are activated. (Criterion 2)

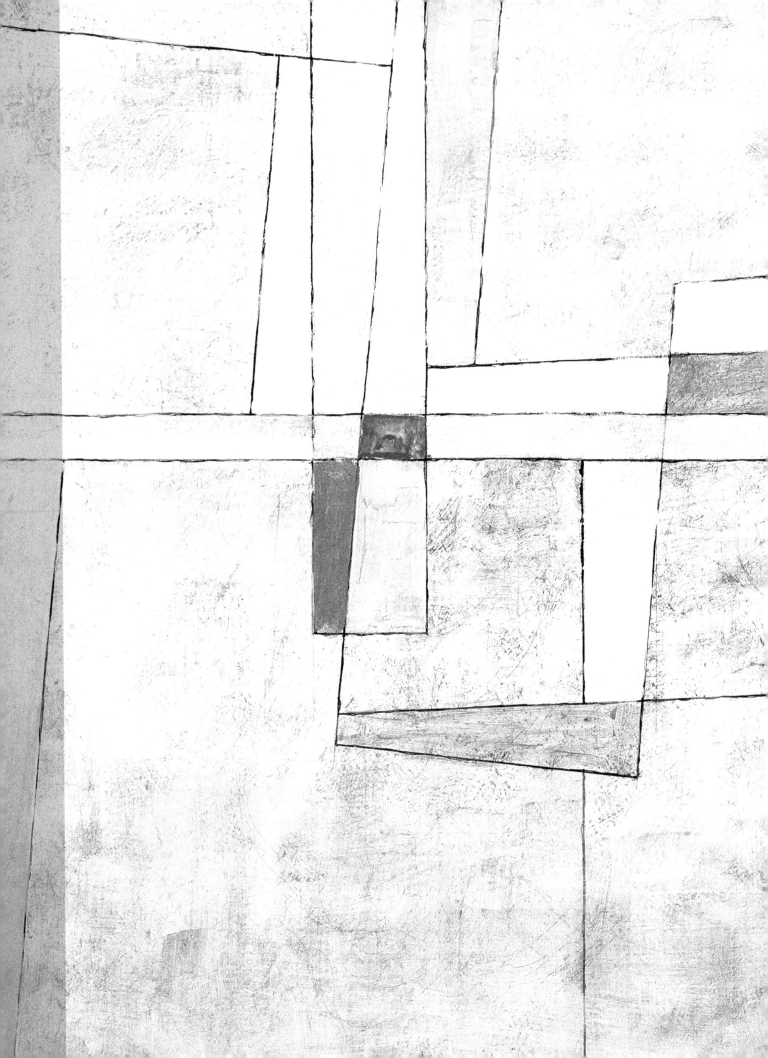

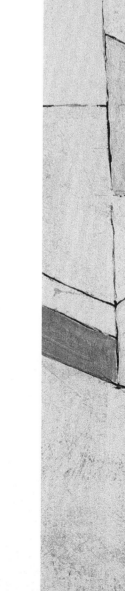

Recognizing the Mode Shifts of the Maladaptive Coping Modes

Preparations for Exercise 6

1. Read the instructions in Chapter 2.

2. Download the Deliberate Practice Reaction Form and Deliberate Practice Diary Form at https://www.apa.org/pubs/books/deliberate-practice-schema-therapy (see the "Clinician and Practitioner Resources" tab; also available in Appendixes A and B, respectively).

Skill Description

Skill Difficulty Level: Intermediate

Maladaptive coping modes are a specific type of schema mode. These modes are triggered to cope with the difficult experiences resulting from activated schemas. For example, a client may "flip" into a maladaptive avoidant coping mode by suddenly detaching from painful schema-triggered emotions. Client markers that signal a possible shift into a maladaptive coping mode include a sudden change in the client's facial expression and tone of voice; rapidly disconnecting emotionally, going quiet, or shrugging; and looking away or suddenly getting angry or frustrated, including at the therapist.

Clients may find it difficult to notice the triggering of their coping modes, or a *mode shift*, because these shifts tend to occur rapidly and largely out of conscious awareness. Thus, therapists often need to draw attention to mode shifts. This exercise focuses on pointing out and inquiring about clients' shifts into a coping mode, as they occur during the session. All client statements in this exercise represent a sudden shift into a maladaptive coping mode (see Appendix C for a full list of maladaptive coping modes). The therapist's responses should draw the client's attention to this shift and inquire about it in an exploratory manner.

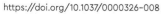

https://doi.org/10.1037/0000326-008
Deliberate Practice in Schema Therapy, by W. T. Behary, J. M. Farrell, A. Vaz, and T. Rousmaniere

> **SKILL CRITERIA FOR EXERCISE 6**
>
> 1. Point out a shift or emotional reaction in the client's behavior.
> 2. Inquire about the client's ability to recognize this shift.
> 3. Raise the possibility that a coping mode has been triggered. (You do not need to identify the specific type of coping mode being triggered.)

Examples of Recognizing the Mode Shifts of the Maladaptive Coping Modes

Example 1

CLIENT: [*Sad*] Yeah, I have been feeling lonelier lately. . . . [*Detached, shift to detached protector mode*] But it's not so important, I don't care. I want to talk about the job interview I have coming up.

THERAPIST: I notice that you start to respond and then you stop and change the subject. (Criterion 1) Are you aware of this? (Criterion 2) It might be your coping mode. (Criterion 3)

Example 2

CLIENT: [*Sad*] I'm still really sad about losing my ex. . . . [*Angry, shift to bully–attack mode*] I don't know why you keep asking me about how I felt when my ex left me. You are starting to sound like a second-rate Dr. Phil.

THERAPIST: I notice that when you become aware of your feelings of pain and hurt, you flip the conversation to tell me about an inadequacy you see in me. (Criterion 1) It is as if you want to distract from your hurt feelings by trying to hurt mine. Are you aware of this? (Criterion 2) Is it possible that a coping mode takes over? (Criterion 3)

Example 3

CLIENT: [*Fearful*] I know you must be getting tired of my complaints and my anger, and I am afraid that you are going to try to transfer me to another therapist. [*Angry, shift to angry protector mode*] Not surprising, really—this is the story of my life. No one really cares. You're just like everyone else. You say you care about me, but you won't keep your promise either. You will just leave me.

THERAPIST: You started telling me about your fears then switched to expressing a lot of anger. (Criterion 1) Are you aware of what just happened? (Criterion 2) I think that a coping mode was triggered to not feel your fears. (Criterion 3)

INSTRUCTIONS FOR EXERCISE 6

Step 1: Role-Play and Feedback

- The client says the first beginner client statement. The therapist improvises a response based on the skill criteria.
- The trainer (or, if not available, the client) provides brief feedback based on the skill criteria.
- The client then repeats the same statement, and the therapist again improvises a response. The trainer (or client) again provides brief feedback.

Step 2: Repeat

- Repeat Step 1 for all the statements in the current difficulty level (beginner, intermediate, or advanced).

Step 3: Assess and Adjust Difficulty

- The therapist completes the Deliberate Practice Reaction Form (see Appendix A) and decides whether to make the exercise easier or harder or to repeat the same difficulty level.

Step 4: Repeat for Approximately 15 Minutes

- Repeat Steps 1 to 3 for at least 15 minutes.
- The trainees then switch therapist and client roles and start over.

> **Now it's your turn! Follow Steps 1 and 2 from the instructions.**

Remember: The goal of the role-play is for trainees to practice improvising responses to the client statements in a manner that (a) uses the skill criteria and (b) feels authentic for the trainee. **Example therapist responses for each client statement are provided at the end of this exercise. Trainees should attempt to improvise their own responses before reading the example responses.**

BEGINNER-LEVEL CLIENT STATEMENTS FOR EXERCISE 6
Beginner Client Statement 1
[Sad] I felt really sad and shed a few tears when my friend called last minute and canceled our plans. **[Upbeat, shift to avoidant protector mode]** I don't know why I am reacting so much; it is really not a big deal at all.
Beginner Client Statement 2
[Angry] I was cheated by not having the opportunity to really know my father. **[Dismissive, shift to angry protector mode]** I didn't really miss anything—he was a jerk.
Beginner Client Statement 3
[Sad] I never felt loved as a child or that I mattered to anyone. **[Disoriented, shift to detached protector mode]** Is that what you asked me about? My mind just went blank.
Beginner Client Statement 4
[Sad] Once again, no one invited me to lunch today. My coworkers make their lunch plans and overlook me like I am invisible. **[Angry, shift to self-aggrandizer mode]** You know what? Who needs them! They are all boring and not very interesting anyway. They are just jealous of me.
Beginner Client Statement 5
[Angry] I feel very angry right now when I think about how little safety I had as a child. It was criminal the way I was treated. **[Flat, shift to detached protector]** I think I am being too sensitive. What doesn't kill you makes you stronger.

> **Assess and adjust the difficulty before moving to the next difficulty level (see Step 3 in the exercise instructions).**

INTERMEDIATE-LEVEL CLIENT STATEMENTS FOR EXERCISE 6

Intermediate Client Statement 1

[Upbeat] I am really looking forward to my friend's party next week. [Hopeless, shift to avoidant protector mode] I don't know why I would think I would have a good time. It isn't worth the effort to get ready and then be disappointed.

Intermediate Client Statement 2

[Neutral] Are you suggesting it was my fault that my girlfriend dumped me because I wasn't meeting all of her needs? [Angry, shift to bully-attack mode] That it's my fault? I am beginning to think that you are not a very good therapist after all.

Intermediate Client Statement 3

[Sad] I have felt really down this month, but suicide? I didn't say anything about suicide. [Angry, shift to bully-attack mode] You must be mixing me up with one of your other clients. Can't you keep us straight? Sharpen up!

Intermediate Client Statement 4

[Anxious] All of a sudden I feel my heart racing and I have a memory of being alone on the playground with the class bully. [Flat, shift to detached protector mode] Wow, that memory just went. I don't know what that was, but it's gone now.

Intermediate Client Statement 5

[Scared] Do you really think you can help me? What is going to happen to me? Will I be alone forever? [Upbeat, shift to approval-seeker mode] But I shouldn't be having these doubts. You are such a good therapist I know you will be able to help me. I am so fortunate that you agreed to work with me.

 Assess and adjust the difficulty before moving to the next difficulty level (see Step 3 in the exercise instructions).

ADVANCED-LEVEL CLIENT STATEMENTS FOR EXERCISE 6

Advanced Client Statement 1

[Positive] I was really looking forward to this session and left early to be on time. [Angry, shift to self-aggrandizer mode] I had a terrible time finding a parking space in your stupid lot. There are obviously not enough spaces for all your clients. I would think that as much as I pay you, you would make sure there was always a space for me.

Advanced Client Statement 2

[Sad] Yeah, I'm still sad about losing my marriage. I still don't understand why it happened. [Angry, shift to bully–attack mode] But I don't know why I have to talk about how I felt when my ex left me. That was long ago, and I don't see what it has to do with anything now. You are starting to sound like a second-rate Dr. Phil.

Advanced Client Statement 3

[Positive] I get a lot out of our sessions. I feel safe here. [Anxious, shift to avoidant protector mode] But maybe I am becoming too dependent on you. Why don't we change our sessions to once a month?

Advanced Client Statement 4

[Anxious] No one can really be counted on, and no one really changes. I don't see the point in looking at the issues from my past. It's just an endless stream of hurts and disappointments. [Flat, shift to perfectionistic overcontroller mode] I am actually fine on my own. I just need to keep working on not needing anyone and doing it all myself. I will be better off.

Advanced Client Statement 5

[Frightened] I had a terrible nightmare last night that the older cousin who sexually abused me was at the door of my house. All day I have felt scared and jumpy. [Flat, shift to detached protector mode] Oh, I'm just being silly. That happened years ago. I have no reason to feel anything about it. No big deal.

 Assess and adjust the difficulty here (see Step 3 in the exercise instructions). If appropriate, follow the instructions to make the exercise even more challenging (see Appendix A).

Example Therapist Responses: Recognizing the Mode Shifts of the Maladaptive Coping Modes

Remember: Trainees should attempt to improvise their own responses before reading the example responses. **Do not read the following responses verbatim unless you are having trouble coming up with your own responses!**

EXAMPLE RESPONSES TO BEGINNER-LEVEL CLIENT STATEMENTS FOR EXERCISE 6
Example Response to Beginner Client Statement 1
I notice that, as you describe how sad you have been feeling, you start to respond and then you stop and start to minimize it. (Criterion 1) Are you aware of doing this? (Criterion 2) It might be your coping mode. (Criterion 3)
Example Response to Beginner Client Statement 2
I notice that you sounded angry for a moment and then switched, dismissing the feelings you shared. (Criterion 1) Are you aware of this shift? (Criterion 2) I think a coping mode was triggered. (Criterion 3)
Example Response to Beginner Client Statement 3
I notice that just after you told me about this painful childhood experience you looked rather blank and a bit confused. (Criterion 1) Are you aware of this? (Criterion 2) It could be that a coping mode was activated. (Criterion 3)
Example Response to Beginner Client Statement 4
I notice that as soon as you started to feel sad you switched to anger and started putting down your coworkers. (Criterion 1) Are you aware of this? (Criterion 2) It sounds to me like a coping mode was triggered. (Criterion 3)
Example Response to Beginner Client Statement 5
Do you notice that when you stop and feel the pain of your childhood you shift very quickly to minimizing it? (Criteria 1 and 2) I think that a coping mode takes over so that you don't feel the pain. (Criterion 3)

EXAMPLE RESPONSES TO INTERMEDIATE-LEVEL CLIENT STATEMENTS FOR EXERCISE 6

Example Response to Intermediate Client Statement 1

You sounded excited about the party and then shifted to hopelessness and pessimism. (Criterion 1) Did you notice that? (Criterion 2) I think that you shifted into a coping mode to protect you from disappointment. (Criterion 3)

Example Response to Intermediate Client Statement 2

Do you notice that you started out being neutral about the breakup and then shifted to feeling angry with me? (Criterion 1) Can you feel that? (Criterion 2) Perhaps it is distracting you from your pain? It feels like a coping mode was triggered. (Criterion 3)

Example Response to Intermediate Client Statement 3

Are you aware of what happened just now? (Criterion 2) You shifted from sounding sad and telling me about your depression to accusing me of being confused and having a poor memory about what you said. (Criterion 1) I think a coping mode was triggered. (Criterion 3)

Example Response to Intermediate Client Statement 4

It sounds like you were aware of a shift in feeling happening. (Criteria 1 and 2) I think you got in touch with an anxiety producing memory, and then a coping mode took over. (Criterion 3)

Example Response to Intermediate Client Statement 5

You started out expressing your fears about being able to get help for your problems in relationships, then you switched to being very complimentary toward me. (Criterion 1) Were you aware of this change? (Criterion 2) I think it could be a coping mode. (Criterion 3)

EXAMPLE RESPONSES TO ADVANCED-LEVEL CLIENT STATEMENTS FOR EXERCISE 6
Example Response to Advanced Client Statement 1
You switched from telling me you were looking forward to our session to being quite angry with me and telling me how special you are, and that you are entitled to special treatment. (Criterion 1) Are you aware of what happened? (Criterion 2) Do you think it could be a coping mode? (Criterion 3)
Example Response to Advanced Client Statement 2
I notice that sometimes when I ask a question that reminds you of your feelings of pain and hurt, you flip to directing anger at me. (Criterion 1) Are you aware of this? (Criterion 2) It seems like a coping mode gets triggered. (Criterion 3)
Example Response to Advanced Client Statement 3
It seems that when you begin to value a relationship and start to feel safe, your fears of depending on anyone get activated and you feel scared. (Criterion 1) Did you notice this shift? (Criterion 2) I think a coping mode was triggered. (Criterion 3)
Example Response to Advanced Client Statement 4
You began expressing some of your fears based on past experience, but as you became upset, you seemed to shift into an action plan instead. (Criterion 1) Are you aware of that happening? (Criterion 2) It looks to me like a coping mode being triggered. (Criterion 3)
Example Response to Advanced Client Statement 5
That nightmare sounds really frightening. Do you notice, however, that you quickly started minimizing those feelings? (Criteria 1 and 2) I think a coping mode was activated. (Criterion 3)

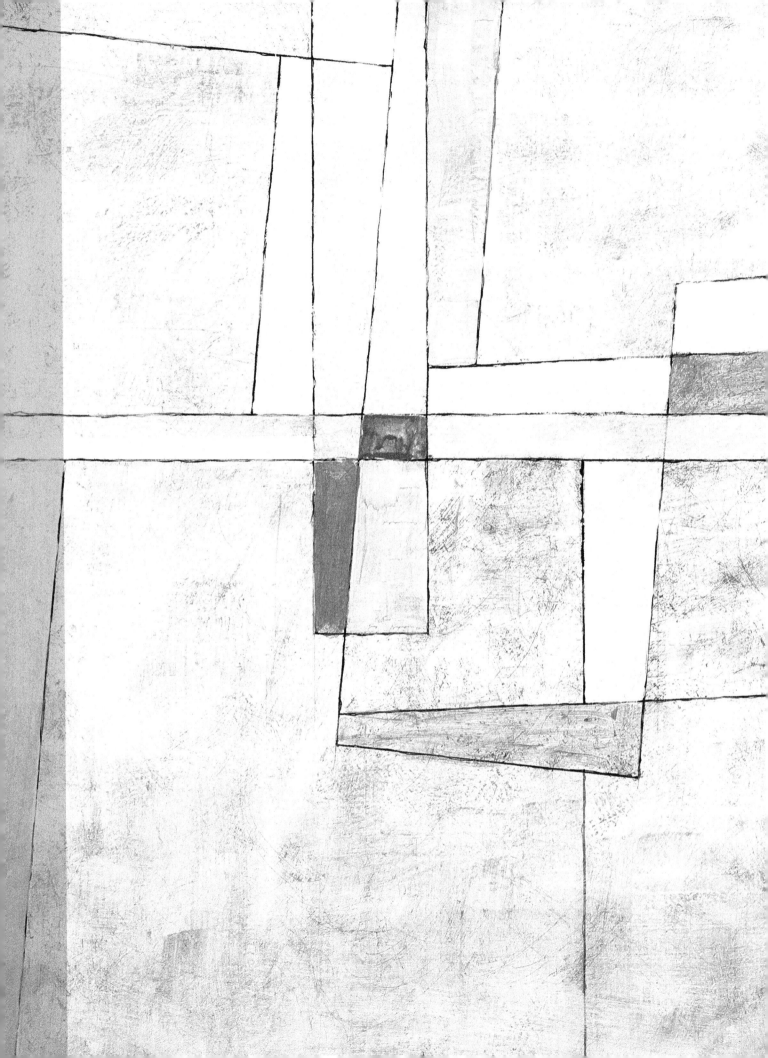

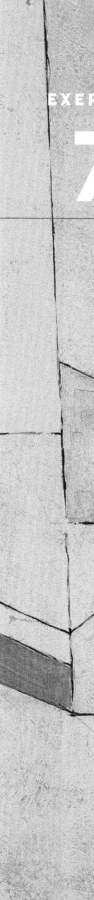

Identifying the Presence of the Demanding/Punitive Inner Critic Mode

Preparations for Exercise 7

1. Read the instructions in Chapter 2.

2. Download the Deliberate Practice Reaction Form and Deliberate Practice Diary Form at https://www.apa.org/pubs/books/deliberate-practice-schema-therapy (see the "Clinician and Practitioner Resources" tab; also available in Appendixes A and B, respectively).

Skill Description

Skill Difficulty Level: Intermediate

The goal of this skill is to identify times when a client makes a self-evaluative comment that reflects their internalized *critic mode*. The activation of the critic mode is made visible by the client's excessive self-criticism and demanding or punitive self-shaming. Clients often develop a dysfunctional inner critic due to the negative judgments and messages they received in childhood from caregivers. For example, when children express a feeling or need and are harshly told "stop whining" or "you'll never amount to anything," it can lead to them having the experience of being "bad" or "wrong." The critic may be primarily demanding or punitive or be a combination of both.

The first step in working with the critic mode is for the therapist to point out the operation of the internalized critic as it occurs. The next step is to begin to inquire about the origins of the critic mode, so that eventually it can be seen as an emotional belief that was internalized in childhood.

https://doi.org/10.1037/0000326-009
Deliberate Practice in Schema Therapy, by W. T. Behary, J. M. Farrell, A. Vaz, and T. Rousmaniere

SKILL CRITERIA FOR EXERCISE 7
1. Point out that the critic mode may be activated.
2. Point out the client's overly demanding or punitive self-criticism.
3. Inquire about the possible origins of the critic mode in childhood and adolescence.

Examples of Identifying the Presence of the Demanding/Punitive Inner Critic Mode

Example 1

CLIENT: [*Hopeless*] I don't know why I expected the date to go well. I should just accept that I am a loser who no one wants to be around. Even my mother didn't particularly like me and said I was a disappointment.

THERAPIST: This sounds like your punitive critic talking now. (Criterion 1) It's a very unfair judgment of you. (Criterion 2) Is it your mother's voice you hear now saying you are a disappointment? (Criterion 3)

Example 2

CLIENT: [*Self-critical*] I have been feeling lonely and sad since the divorce, but I know I am making a big deal of it and acting like a whiner. I should just be able to close the chapter and get on with my life.

THERAPIST: That last statement is really harsh and unreasonable. (Criterion 2) It sounds like your critic mode to me. (Criterion 1) Who in your childhood would have referred to you as a whiner when you felt sad? (Criterion 3)

Example 3

CLIENT: [*Anxious*] I am so afraid that I will also drive you away, just like everyone else in my life. You must be so fed up with me. I know I have made some progress, but I don't try hard enough. All I do is whine about my life. I don't do anything about it. I am sick of myself.

THERAPIST: I think your critic mode might be triggered. (Criterion 1) You started telling me about your fear, also realizing that you have made progress, then ended with being overly critical of yourself. (Criterion 2) What experiences in your life caused you to have such a negative opinion of yourself? (Criterion 3)

INSTRUCTIONS FOR EXERCISE 7

Step 1: Role-Play and Feedback

- The client says the first beginner client statement. The therapist improvises a response based on the skill criteria.
- The trainer (or, if not available, the client) provides brief feedback based on the skill criteria.
- The client then repeats the same statement, and the therapist again improvises a response. The trainer (or client) again provides brief feedback.

Step 2: Repeat

- Repeat Step 1 for all the statements in the current difficulty level (beginner, intermediate, or advanced).

Step 3: Assess and Adjust Difficulty

- The therapist completes the Deliberate Practice Reaction Form (see Appendix A) and decides whether to make the exercise easier or harder or to repeat the same difficulty level.

Step 4: Repeat for Approximately 15 Minutes

- Repeat Steps 1 to 3 for at least 15 minutes.
- The trainees then switch therapist and client roles and start over.

Now it's your turn! Follow Steps 1 and 2 from the instructions.

Remember: The goal of the role-play is for trainees to practice improvising responses to the client statements in a manner that (a) uses the skill criteria and (b) feels authentic for the trainee. **Example therapist responses for each client statement are provided at the end of this exercise. Trainees should attempt to improvise their own responses before reading the example responses.**

BEGINNER-LEVEL CLIENT STATEMENTS FOR EXERCISE 7
Beginner Client Statement 1
[Sad] You are very nice and caring to me, but that's because you're a therapist. That's what you are supposed to do. I cannot imagine how anyone in the real world would want to put up with me if they really knew me. I am such a pathetic loser.
Beginner Client Statement 2
[Fearful] I don't know how I am ever going to give this presentation in front of the committee. I have prepared and prepared for months, but I know it's not enough. I'll never be as entertaining as my colleagues. I am going to make a fool of myself.
Beginner Client Statement 3
[Sad] I was so hoping that maybe he would ask me to join him for dinner. I thought we were making a good connection. What an idiot I am! What was I thinking? I am so ugly and boring. Why would a good-looking, charming, and intelligent guy like that want to date someone like me?
Beginner Client Statement 4
[Anxious] I'm sorry. I know you are doing your best to help me. It must be so frustrating for you having to deal with someone like me. I don't follow through on anything. All I do is complain. I am destined to be stuck in an unhappy life and it's all my fault. I really cannot stand myself anymore!
Beginner Client Statement 5
[Self-critical] I am afraid to tell you that I was drinking again this weekend. I know that you will be angry with me. I deserve to be punished. I am so weak and incapable of keeping any commitments. My father was right. I will never amount to anything.

 Assess and adjust the difficulty before moving to the next difficulty level (see Step 3 in the exercise instructions).

INTERMEDIATE-LEVEL CLIENT STATEMENTS FOR EXERCISE 7
Intermediate Client Statement 1
[Disgusted] I can't believe I was given a promotion at work. I'm such a fraud. I bet they'll figure out that I'm incompetent, and they'll probably take away the promotion. It's gonna be so embarrassing.
Intermediate Client Statement 2
[Sad/inconsolable] Of course he cheated on me. Look at me . . . I don't take care of myself. I don't appreciate him enough. I am always complaining. I don't satisfy him sexually. He is completely turned off by me, and it's all my fault.
Intermediate Client Statement 3
[Quiet/anxious] I didn't fill out the inventory you asked me to do. I know I am difficult and distracted; I cannot remember things and I make excuses. You're probably going to be sorry you agreed to work with me.
Intermediate Client Statement 4
[Angry/disgusted] I feel very angry right now and I have no right to feel this way. I am the one who destroys my friendships. I push people away. I am too sensitive and demanding and needy. I cry too easily and expect everyone to feel sorry for me; how pathetic! My mother was right. I am damaged goods.
Intermediate Client Statement 5
[Hopeless/disgusted] Why can I never get it right? I lost another sale this week, and my boss was clearly disappointed. I can't blame him. I am not working hard enough. I know my associate would have done a much better job securing this sale. I am not clever enough.

 Assess and adjust the difficulty before moving to the next difficulty level (see Step 3 in the exercise instructions).

ADVANCED-LEVEL CLIENT STATEMENTS FOR EXERCISE 7
Advanced Client Statement 1
[Angry] You probably don't believe me, but I was really looking forward to this session. If I was smart enough, I would have left my house a little early to avoid the traffic. But I am so stupid, and I didn't pay attention to the time again, and now I'm late. I yelled at myself the whole way here. I am tired of being me.
Advanced Client Statement 2
[Sad] I don't deserve to be happy. It's my fault that my mother is lonely all the time. I'm selfish. I should be living with her and keeping her company. If something happens to her, she says I'll live to regret my actions. She's probably right about that too.
Advanced Client Statement 3
[Angry] I'm just not good enough. I failed one part of my licensing exam again and will have to take it over. I just don't have what it takes to be a doctor. My father told me I should not try to take on such a difficult job—that it was beyond me.
Advanced Client Statement 4
[Regretful] I have spent so many years in therapy. What is wrong with me? How could it take so long to realize that I was living in a destructive relationship? Why didn't I see it sooner? Maybe I liked being mistreated. Perhaps I am just a drama queen looking for attention. My mother was right. What a waste of time. I'll never forgive myself.
Advanced Client Statement 5
[Frightened] I got as far as the parking lot and I froze. I couldn't get myself to walk into the restaurant. When am I going to grow up and get over this ridiculous phobia? I act like a weak little pathetic child who is afraid of ghosts. I'm an embarrassment.

> Assess and adjust the difficulty here (see Step 3 in the exercise instructions). If appropriate, follow the instructions to make the exercise even more challenging (see Appendix A).

Example Therapist Responses: Identifying the Presence of the Demanding/Punitive Inner Critic Mode

Remember: Trainees should attempt to improvise their own responses before reading the example responses. **Do not read the following responses verbatim unless you are having trouble coming up with your own responses!**

EXAMPLE RESPONSES TO BEGINNER-LEVEL CLIENT STATEMENTS FOR EXERCISE 7
Example Response to Beginner Client Statement 1
This sounds like your critic mode, (Criterion 1) the part of you that becomes unfairly harsh and shaming toward yourself. (Criterion 2) What early experiences do you think led to such a negative view of yourself? (Criterion 3)
Example Response to Beginner Client Statement 2
I am detecting the voice of your internal critic mode. (Criterion 1) Nothing is ever good enough for this critic. (Criterion 1) Where did you learn such an unrelenting standard? (Criterion 3)
Example Response to Beginner Client Statement 3
Feels like you are speaking from your critic mode now, (Criterion 1) and the message is harsh and terribly unfair. (Criterion 2) Where could that voice come from? (Criterion 3)
Example Response to Beginner Client Statement 4
This sounds like your critic mode speaking right now, (Criterion 1) the one that immediately puts you down and is punitive when you are not perfect. (Criterion 2) I wonder what earlier experiences in your life led to the development of this critic mode. (Criterion 3)
Example Response to Beginner Client Statement 5
I hear the critic mode being triggered right now. (Criterion 1) I guess this was what you learned from your father and now it lives inside of you? (Criterion 3) However, that internal critic is really unreasonable and punitive. (Criterion 2)

EXAMPLE RESPONSES TO INTERMEDIATE-LEVEL CLIENT STATEMENTS FOR EXERCISE 7
Example Response to Intermediate Client Statement 1
Those negative statements are incredibly harsh and critical. (Criterion 2) They sound like the critic mode to me. (Criterion 1) Who earlier in your life gave you the message that you were lazy and stupid and that you could never work hard enough? (Criterion 3)
Example Response to Intermediate Client Statement 2
That is a completely unfair evaluation of you. (Criterion 2) It comes from your internal critic (Criterion 1) and is just not accurate. Where did you learn to blame yourself for anything that goes wrong? (Criterion 3)
Example Response to Intermediate Client Statement 3
I hear your critic mode. (Criterion 1) Your evaluation of yourself is in absolutes that are excessively demanding. (Criterion 2) I wonder whose voice that is? (Criterion 3)
Example Response to Intermediate Client Statement 4
We are hearing your critic mode right now. (Criterion 1) Calling yourself "damaged goods" is very punitive. (Criterion 2) Whose voice are you hearing right now? (Criterion 3)
Example Response to Intermediate Client Statement 5
Wait a minute—your critic (Criterion 1) is exaggerating the situation and only seeing the negative, as usual. (Criterion 2) Where did you learn to be so demanding and critical of yourself? (Criterion 3)

EXAMPLE RESPONSES TO ADVANCED-LEVEL CLIENT STATEMENTS FOR EXERCISE 7
Example Response to Advanced Client Statement 1
It is way too extreme to call yourself "stupid" for not knowing how busy the traffic would be. (Criterion 2) That statement is a good example of your critic mode in action. (Criterion 1) Who in your early life was so demanding and shaming? (Criterion 3)
Example Response to Advanced Client Statement 2
Wow, those messages don't leave any room for you to be happy—as if your life was only for taking care of your mother. (Criterion 2) That view sounds like your critic mode to me. (Criterion 1) Is it your mother's voice you are hearing? (Criterion 3)
Example Response to Advanced Client Statement 3
I have to stop your critic mode right there. (Criterion 1) You failed only one part of the exam, but that is all that your critic focuses on. It does not mean that you cannot be a doctor. (Criterion 2) Your father's evaluation was unfair and overly negative, and now your critic is echoing him. (Criterion 3)
Example Response to Advanced Client Statement 4
Wow! I hear your critic loud and clear in those messages! (Criterion 1) Your critic's statements are very harsh and unfair to you. (Criterion 2) It sounds like you are hearing your mother's voice calling you a "drama queen." (Criterion 3)
Example Response to Advanced Client Statement 5
We are hearing your critic mode now, (Criterion 1) and it is not helpful or accurate. (Criterion 2) Where did you learn to judge your feelings so harshly? (Criterion 3)

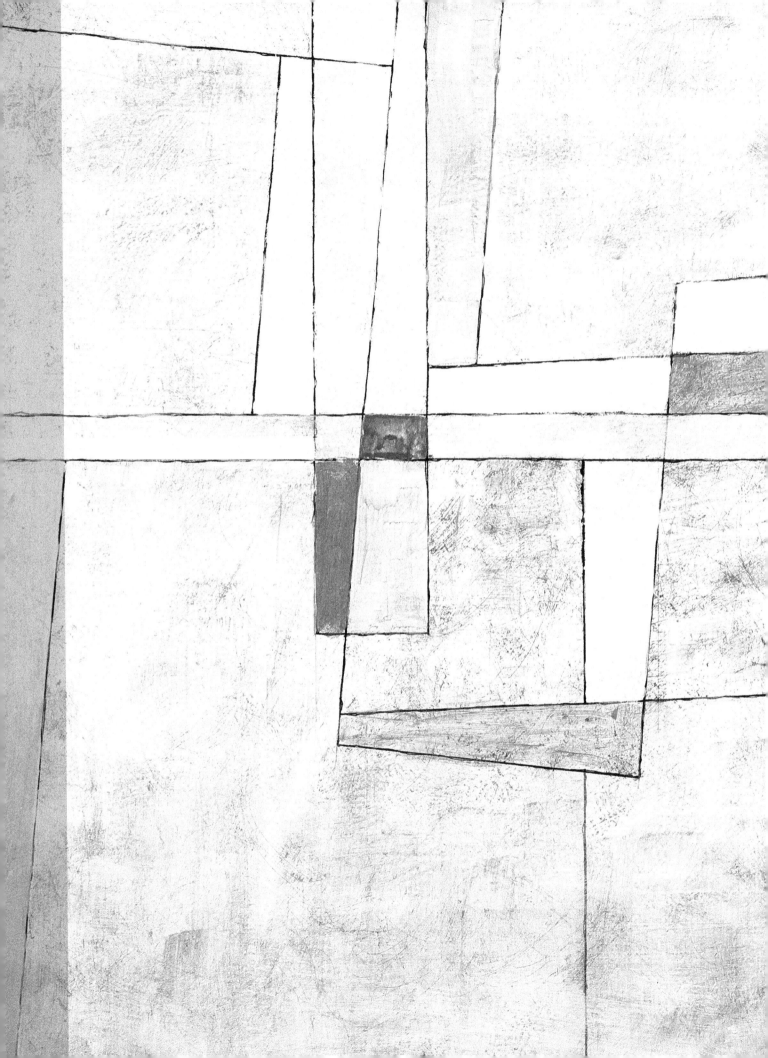

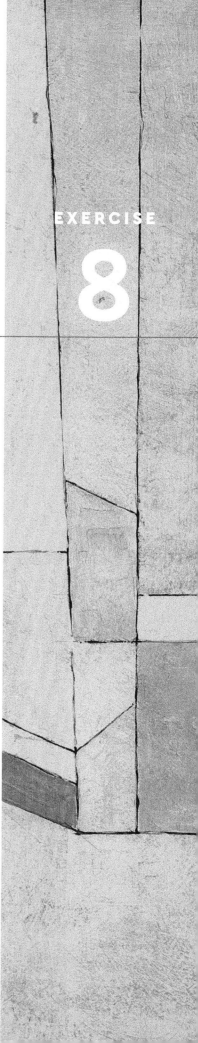

Identifying the Presence of the Angry and Vulnerable Child Modes

Preparations for Exercise 8

1. Read the instructions in Chapter 2.

2. Download the Deliberate Practice Reaction Form and Deliberate Practice Diary Form at https://www.apa.org/pubs/books/deliberate-practice-schema-therapy (see the "Clinician and Practitioner Resources" tab; also available in Appendixes A and B, respectively).

Skill Description

Skill Difficulty Level: Intermediate

A core skill for schema therapists is identifying angry and vulnerable child modes. These are times when a client appears to experience an emotional state that is either too intense for the present moment in adult life or has a childlike, helpless quality that relates to a core childhood need that was not met or only partially not met. These modes are developed in childhood as a result of caregiving that was dismissive or absent.

Angry and vulnerable child modes can be identified in therapy through changes in the client's emotional intensity, bodily posture, tone, and language. In the angry child mode, the client presents with anger that seems childlike, even approaching a tantrum, with statements such as "it's not fair" and "you don't hear me." In the vulnerable child mode, the client presents as helpless, often experiencing intense fear, sadness, or loneliness.

This exercise focuses on the first step in working with the child modes, which is to point out their presence, with the goal of helping the client understand these reactions as occurring due to childhood experiences with caregivers. Throughout this exercise, the therapist should strive to use a gentle, warm, and tentative tone, making sure not to assume that the client is already aware of their emotional state and triggered child mode. The therapist may also occasionally lean forward to add emphasis to the intervention.

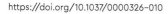

https://doi.org/10.1037/0000326-010
Deliberate Practice in Schema Therapy, by W. T. Behary, J. M. Farrell, A. Vaz, and T. Rousmaniere

---

SKILL CRITERIA FOR EXERCISE 8

1. Gently point out the client's emotional intensity.
2. Inquire about the client's ability to recognize this emotional state.
3. Raise the possibility that this emotional state represents the triggering of an angry or vulnerable child mode.

Examples of Identifying the Presence of the Angry and Vulnerable Child Modes

Example 1

CLIENT: [*Upset*] It's just so hard to believe that my best friend of 30 years is really moving so far away next month. I cannot imagine how I will get on with my life without her steady support. It's like my dad leaving us all those years ago.

THERAPIST: I notice that you are becoming upset as you describe this to me. (Criterion 1) Are you aware of this shift in yourself too? (Criterion 2) I wonder if this might be your vulnerable child mode getting triggered because of the activation of a schema in this situation? (Criterion 3)

Example 2

CLIENT: [*Angry*] I know you say that you care about me, but how can I believe it? I mean why would I believe anyone could really care when my own mother never paid any attention to me? You are just my therapist.

THERAPIST: You seem to be getting a little angry and upset. (Criterion 1) Can you notice the shift into the angry part of you right now? (Criterion 2) I wonder if the angry child mode might be getting triggered remembering how little love you had as a child. (Criterion 3)

Example 3

CLIENT: [*Hopeless*] I was just remembering how my coworkers laughed outside my office again yesterday. I suspect they were making jokes about me. I am always the target of jokes and criticism. It's the story of my life. Never ends.

THERAPIST: I see that when you recall this event, you seem to shift into a sad and hopeless state. (Criterion 1) I wonder if you can feel that part of you getting triggered right now? (Criterion 2) Maybe "little you," your vulnerable child mode, is being triggered in this situation? (Criterion 3)

INSTRUCTIONS FOR EXERCISE 8

Step 1: Role-Play and Feedback

- The client says the first beginner client statement. The therapist improvises a response based on the skill criteria.
- The trainer (or, if not available, the client) provides brief feedback based on the skill criteria.
- The client then repeats the same statement, and the therapist again improvises a response. The trainer (or client) again provides brief feedback.

Step 2: Repeat

- Repeat Step 1 for all the statements in the current difficulty level (beginner, intermediate, or advanced).

Step 3: Assess and Adjust Difficulty

- The therapist completes the Deliberate Practice Reaction Form (see Appendix A) and decides whether to make the exercise easier or harder or to repeat the same difficulty level.

Step 4: Repeat for Approximately 15 Minutes

- Repeat Steps 1 to 3 for at least 15 minutes.
- The trainees then switch therapist and client roles and start over.

> **Now it's your turn! Follow Steps 1 and 2 from the instructions.**

Remember: The goal of the role-play is for trainees to practice improvising responses to the client statements in a manner that (a) uses the skill criteria and (b) feels authentic for the trainee. **Example therapist responses for each client statement are provided at the end of this exercise. Trainees should attempt to improvise their own responses before reading the example responses.**

BEGINNER-LEVEL CLIENT STATEMENTS FOR EXERCISE 8
Beginner Client Statement 1
[Desperate] I waited all weekend for him to call me. His rejection is so unbearable. I am never going to find someone to love me. I will be alone forever.
Beginner Client Statement 2
[Devastated] My husband speaks to his cousin every day and barely says good morning to me. I don't matter to him. I don't matter to anyone.
Beginner Client Statement 3
[Anxious] You look like you're getting tired of me just like everyone else. I can't blame you. I drive everyone away from me eventually. I just can't bear to lose you too.
Beginner Client Statement 4
[Sad] It's just so hard to believe that my best friend of 30 years is really moving so far away next month. I cannot imagine how I will get on with my life without her steady support. It's like my dad leaving us all those years ago.
Beginner Client Statement 5
[Hopeless] I was just remembering how my coworkers laughed outside my office again yesterday. I suspect they were making jokes about me. I am always the target of jokes and criticism. It's the story of my life. Never ends.

 Assess and adjust the difficulty before moving to the next difficulty level (see Step 3 in the exercise instructions).

INTERMEDIATE-LEVEL CLIENT STATEMENTS FOR EXERCISE 8
Intermediate Client Statement 1
[Angry] There is no such thing as a "safe place." I never had any protection as a child. It was criminal the way I was treated. It's amazing I survived. It was so unfair! My parents should be in jail.
Intermediate Client Statement 2
[Hopeless] Once again, my coworker canceled our lunch date. I wish you would just accept that there is no hope for me to make friends or have an intimate connection with anyone. It's never going to happen. My own mother didn't play with me or even talk to me, let alone show me any love or affection.
Intermediate Client Statement 3
[Angry] So, you're really going to take a vacation when I am in such a state of chaos?! You're just like everyone else! Just admit it—you really need to get away from me. I can't count on anyone; never could and never will.
Intermediate Client Statement 4
[Overwhelmed] I can't do it! I cannot attend this business event. I know I will be standing in a corner all by myself. No one will talk to me, they will look right past me, they will probably be talking about me with each other. It will be like primary school all over again.
Intermediate Client Statement 5
[Devastated] I will never be happy. The divorce has ruined me forever. I am a forgettable person, it's the story of my life. Certainly, my dad felt this way when he left my mom and me when I was little. It's exactly the same.

 Assess and adjust the difficulty before moving to the next difficulty level (see Step 3 in the exercise instructions).

ADVANCED-LEVEL CLIENT STATEMENTS FOR EXERCISE 8

Advanced Client Statement 1

[Frightened] I had a terrible nightmare last night that the older cousin who sexually abused me was at the door of my house. I was in a panic. I can't believe this still haunts me. I can't take it anymore.

Advanced Client Statement 2

[Angry] She is forever making promises she doesn't keep! I know she just had a baby and is in the middle of moving, but when I send her a message and she doesn't respond for almost an hour, it's outrageous! She was always the golden child—the one my parents favored. She gets away with everything. I'm sick of this; it's just not fair! I'm not speaking to her anymore, and I will not be helping her with her new baby.

Advanced Client Statement 3

[Despairing] How can I possibly make challenging life decisions for myself? Every decision, big or small, was always made by my mother. Now, she's drunk all the time, or sick in bed, and I don't know what to do. I don't know how to take care of myself. I will never figure it out. It's too hard.

Advanced Client Statement 4

[Angry] I am so tired of being the target of my family's jokes and criticism. I have always been the scapegoat. They did it to me again last week at my cousin's wedding when someone made the toast and shared a story that they knew would embarrass me! No one thinks about my feelings, no one cares. I hate them all.

Advanced Client Statement 5

[Sad and angry] I can't believe that you forgot the name of my neighbor who abused me! How could you forget?! Am I not important to you? Are you just like everyone else who pretends to listen but really ignores me? You say you care, but you're a liar. Everyone lies to me.

 Assess and adjust the difficulty here (see Step 3 in the exercise instructions). If appropriate, follow the instructions to make the exercise even more challenging (see Appendix A).

Example Therapist Responses: Identifying the Presence of the Angry and Vulnerable Child Modes

Remember: Trainees should attempt to improvise their own responses before reading the example responses. **Do not read the following responses verbatim unless you are having trouble coming up with your own responses!**

EXAMPLE RESPONSES TO BEGINNER-LEVEL CLIENT STATEMENTS FOR EXERCISE 8
Example Response to Beginner Client Statement 1
I notice you are becoming extremely sad as you tell me this. (Criterion 1) Are you aware of the shift in yourself right now? (Criterion 2) Perhaps this is your vulnerable child mode getting triggered as you feel the activation of a schema linked with that fear of aloneness. (Criterion 3)
Example Response to Beginner Client Statement 2
I notice that you seemed to shift into a very deep and intense sadness. (Criterion 1) Are you aware of this shift in yourself? (Criterion 2) Perhaps this is your vulnerable child mode showing up, as a schema gets activated, mirroring a way you have felt since you were little? (Criterion 3)
Example Response to Beginner Client Statement 3
Sounds like you are experiencing some intense feelings regarding our connection and my caring for you. (Criterion 1) Are you aware of this shift happening in yourself right now? (Criterion 2) Maybe this is your vulnerable child mode getting triggered by a schema, losing the people you needed the most when you were little. (Criterion 3)
Example Response to Beginner Client Statement 4
I notice that you are becoming sad and even desperate as you describe this to me. (Criterion 1) Are you aware of this shift in yourself too? (Criterion 2) I wonder if this might be your vulnerable child mode getting triggered because of the activation of a schema in this situation? (Criterion 3)
Example Response to Beginner Client Statement 5
I see that when you recall this event you seem to shift into a sad and hopeless state. (Criterion 1) I wonder if you can feel that part of you getting triggered right now? (Criterion 2) Maybe "little you," your vulnerable child mode, is being triggered in this situation? (Criterion 3)

EXAMPLE RESPONSES TO INTERMEDIATE-LEVEL CLIENT STATEMENTS FOR EXERCISE 8

Example Response to Intermediate Client Statement 1

I notice a shift to a state of intense anger as you speak about this. (Criterion 1) Are you aware of this shift in yourself? (Criterion 2) Has "little you," the angry child mode, been triggered? The voice inside you who is enraged when triggered, recalling the injustices that you felt when you were helpless and powerless. (Criterion 3)

Example Response to Intermediate Client Statement 2

I am sensing a hopeless state in you as you speak of this event. (Criterion 1) Can you sense this in yourself right now? (Criterion 2) Perhaps your vulnerable child mode is activated as you feel the power of schema taking you back to your own mother's neglectful ways. (Criterion 3)

Example Response to Intermediate Client Statement 3

You are shifting into a very strong emotional state right now. (Criterion 1) Can you feel it? (Criterion 2) Your angry child is feeling blamed and forgotten again, and it feels like another injustice just like when you were a child. (Criterion 3)

Example Response to Intermediate Client Statement 4

I am sensing a shift in your emotional state. (Criterion 1) Can you sense it too? (Criterion 2) Perhaps this is your frightened vulnerable child mode, when a schema is activated, expecting to be treated the same way you did back then. (Criterion 3)

Example Response to Intermediate Client Statement 5

Feels like an intense shift in your emotional state as you look at the aftermath of your divorce. (Criterion 1) I sense you are aware of this shift, (Criterion 2) as you make the link to your experiences with your dad and his absence in your life. This feels like your vulnerable child mode is getting triggered. (Criterion 3)

EXAMPLE RESPONSES TO ADVANCED-LEVEL CLIENT STATEMENTS FOR EXERCISE 8

Example Response to Advanced Client Statement 1

I can see that, as you recall this terrible event in your life, you seem to shift into an intense emotional state. (Criterion 1) I suspect you are noticing it too? (Criterion 2) Is your vulnerable child mode getting triggered? And when it does, the threat becomes overwhelmingly real and the danger feels very present. (Criterion 3)

Example Response to Advanced Client Statement 2

I see how upset you feel that your sister is letting you down. You seem to be shifting into a strong state of anger. (Criterion 1) Can you sense the escalation happening inside of you? (Criterion 2) This is your angry child mode getting triggered as schemas get activated, reminding you of always being in the shadows while your sister enjoyed preferential treatment. It carries a strong memory of unfairness. (Criterion 3)

Example Response to Advanced Client Statement 3

I hear a shift in your tone and your words to one of hopelessness and perhaps despair. (Criterion 1) Do you notice yourself shifting right now? (Criterion 2) This is probably your vulnerable child mode getting triggered as your schemas are getting activated during an important decision-making time in your life. (Criterion 3)

Example Response to Advanced Client Statement 4

I notice a shift as you tell the story, to feeling intensely angry and perhaps hurt. (Criterion 1) Can you sense that shift too? (Criterion 2) Feels like an angry child mode, that little part of you who has shown up to remind us that she is tired of feeling used and humiliated. (Criterion 3)

Example Response to Advanced Client Statement 5

I see an intense shift in your emotional state, to one that is angry, hurt, and very upset. (Criterion 1) Can you sense this part of you too? (Criterion 2) I see this as the vulnerable and angry child modes, the little parts of you that are incredibly sad and hurt and angry when it feels just like it did when you were young and treated as if you don't matter. This part is really furious and tired of being treated this way. (Criterion 3)

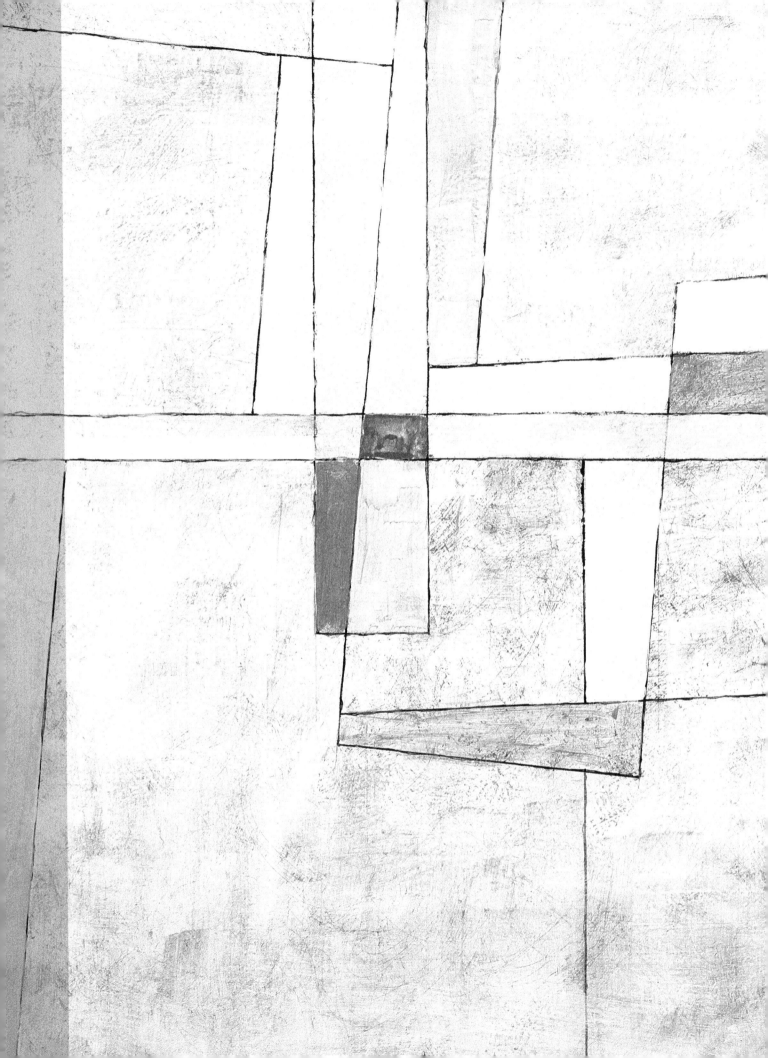

Limited Reparenting for the Angry and Vulnerable Child Modes

Preparations for Exercise 9

1. Read the instructions in Chapter 2.

2. Download the Deliberate Practice Reaction Form and Deliberate Practice Diary Form at https://www.apa.org/pubs/books/deliberate-practice-schema-therapy (see the "Clinician and Practitioner Resources" tab; also available in Appendixes A and B, respectively).

Skill Description

Skill Difficulty Level: Advanced

The schema therapy (ST) view is that clients are often understandably "needy" based on the experience of core childhood needs not being met. Limited reparenting includes a therapist in the role of a "good parent," offering empathy in facial expression, body posture, vocal awareness, and word crafting, all designed to convey support and healing messages of acceptance, connection, frustration tolerance, guidance, safety, and autonomy. It is one of the core ST interventions employed to provide the client with a corrective emotional experience of having the unmet need that is present in the child mode met within the limits of the therapy relationship. The core childhood needs that are addressed in ST through limited reparenting are as follows:

- secure attachment to others, including safety, stability, nurturance and acceptance
- autonomy, competence, and sense of identity
- freedom to express valid needs and emotions
- spontaneity and play
- realistic limits and self-control

https://doi.org/10.1037/0000326-011

Deliberate Practice in Schema Therapy, by W. T. Behary, J. M. Farrell, A. Vaz, and T. Rousmaniere

Limited reparenting in schema therapy involves the therapist's overall style as well as their actions. For this exercise, the therapist improvises a response to each client statement following these skill criteria:

1. Validate the client's feelings and normalize within the client's unmet needs in childhood and adolescence. Clients will often not be explicit about their early needs that were not adequately met. In these cases, the therapist tentatively suggests an unmet need that would make sense given the client's statement.

2. Act to meet the client's present needs. Although there are many actions a schema therapist can take, in this exercise we focus on a limited number of actions:
   - reminding the client of your connection and support
   - encouraging client's emotional expression
   - suggesting an imagery exercise that meets the need (e.g., safe place imagery)

For each intervention, the therapist presents one of these actions in a warm, tentative tone.

SKILL CRITERIA FOR EXERCISE 9

1. Validate the client's emotional expression and triggering of their child mode as understandable given their early unmet needs.
2. Take one of the following actions to meet the need within professional boundaries:
   Action 1: Remind the client of your connection and support.
   Action 2: Encourage the client's emotional expression.
   Action 3: Suggest an imagery exercise that meets the need.

Examples of Limited Reparenting for the Angry and Vulnerable Child Modes

Example 1

CLIENT: [*Upset*] It's just so hard to believe that my best friend of 30 years is really moving so far away next month. I cannot imagine how I will get on with my life without her steady support. It's like my dad leaving us all those years ago.

THERAPIST: It makes sense that your vulnerable part is expressing herself here as you remember the loss of your dad. Her hurts and her fears are understandable given that you had little support for emotional expression as a child. (Criterion 1) We need to be kind and patient with this part of you. Can we focus right now on our connection? This is a place to give "little you" the support she needs. (Criterion 2, Action 1)

Example 2

CLIENT: [*Angry*] I know you say that you care about me, but how can I believe it? I mean why would I believe anyone could really care when my own mother never paid any attention to me? The moment I expressed any anger she shut me down or left.

THERAPIST: Of course you wouldn't trust my words. That makes sense to me, as the vulnerable part of you had no one to count on. No one showed any consistent caring for you, and you could not safely express your anger as a little child. It will take you time to have confidence in my caring. (Criterion 1) I welcome your expression of anger. Is there more anger you might want to express? (Criterion 2, Action 2)

Example 3

CLIENT: [*Sad*] I was just remembering how my coworkers laughed outside my office again yesterday. I suspect they were making jokes about me. I was always the target of jokes and criticism when I was a kid. It's the story of my life. It never ends.

THERAPIST: It must be so hard for that vulnerable part of you when he senses that he is becoming the target of bullies again. As a child he had no protection or safety, and he surely needed that. (Criterion 1) Let's see if we can bring some protection and comfort to this part of you now using safety imagery. Perhaps you might close your eyes and take a moment to see and sense him? I will guide you. (Criterion 2, Action 3)

INSTRUCTIONS FOR EXERCISE 9

Step 1: Role-Play and Feedback

- The client says the first beginner client statement. The therapist improvises a response based on the skill criteria.
- The trainer (or, if not available, the client) provides brief feedback based on the skill criteria.
- The client then repeats the same statement, and the therapist again improvises a response. The trainer (or client) again provides brief feedback.

Step 2: Repeat

- Repeat Step 1 for all the statements in the current difficulty level (beginner, intermediate, or advanced).

Step 3: Assess and Adjust Difficulty

- The therapist completes the Deliberate Practice Reaction Form (see Appendix A) and decides whether to make the exercise easier or harder or to repeat the same difficulty level.

Step 4: Repeat for Approximately 15 Minutes

- Repeat Steps 1 to 3 for at least 15 minutes.
- The trainees then switch therapist and client roles and start over.

Now it's your turn! Follow Steps 1 and 2 from the instructions.

Remember: The goal of the role-play is for trainees to practice improvising responses to the client statements in a manner that (a) uses the skill criteria and (b) feels authentic for the trainee. **Example therapist responses for each client statement are provided at the end of this exercise. Trainees should attempt to improvise their own responses before reading the example responses.**

BEGINNER-LEVEL CLIENT STATEMENTS FOR EXERCISE 9
Beginner Client Statement 1
[Sad] I waited all weekend for him to call me. His rejection is so unbearable. I am never going to find someone to love me. I will be alone forever.
Beginner Client Statement 2
[Devastated] My partner speaks to his cousin every day and barely says good morning to me. I don't matter to him. I don't matter to anyone. I am invisible. No one would notice if I fell off the face of the earth.
Beginner Client Statement 3
[Nervous] You look like you're getting tired of me just like everyone else. I can't blame you. I drive everyone away from me eventually. I just can't bear to lose you too.
Beginner Client Statement 4
[Upset] It's just so hard to believe that my best friend of 30 years is really moving so far away next month. I cannot imagine how I will get on with my life without her steady support. It's like my dad leaving us all those years ago.
Beginner Client Statement 5
[Hopeless] I was just remembering how my coworkers laughed outside my office again yesterday. I suspect they were making jokes about me. I am always the target of jokes and criticism. It's the story of my life. It never ends.

 Assess and adjust the difficulty before moving to the next difficulty level (see Step 3 in the exercise instructions).

INTERMEDIATE-LEVEL CLIENT STATEMENTS FOR EXERCISE 9

Intermediate Client Statement 1

[Angry] There is no such thing as a "safe place." I never had any protection as a child. It was criminal the way I was treated. It's amazing I survived. It was so unfair! My parents should be in jail.

Intermediate Client Statement 2

[Hopeless] Once again, my coworker canceled our lunch date. I wish you would just accept that there is no hope for me to make friends or have an intimate connection with anyone. It's never going to happen. My own mother didn't play with me or even talk to me, let alone show me any love or affection.

Intermediate Client Statement 3

[Angry] I know you say that you care about me, but how can I believe it? I mean, why would I believe anyone could really care when my own mother never paid any attention to me? The moment I expressed any anger she shut me down or left.

Intermediate Client Statement 4

[Overwhelmed] I can't do it! I can't attend this business event. I know I'll be standing in a corner all by myself. No one will talk to me; they'll look right past me. They'll probably be talking about me with each other. It will be like primary school all over again.

Intermediate Client Statement 5

[Devastated] I will never be happy. The divorce has ruined me forever. I am a forgettable person—it's the story of my life. Certainly, my dad felt this way when he left my mom and me when I was little. It's exactly the same.

 Assess and adjust the difficulty before moving to the next difficulty level (see Step 3 in the exercise instructions).

ADVANCED-LEVEL CLIENT STATEMENTS FOR EXERCISE 9
Advanced Client Statement 1
[Frightened] I had a terrible nightmare last night that the older cousin who sexually abused me was at the door of my house. I was in a panic. I can't believe this still haunts me. I can't take it anymore.
Advanced Client Statement 2
[Angry] She is forever making promises she does not keep! I know she just had a baby and is in the middle of moving, but when I send her a message and she doesn't respond for almost an hour, it's outrageous! She was always the golden child, the one my parents favored. She gets away with everything. I'm sick of this; it's just not fair! I'm not speaking to her anymore, and I will not be helping her with her new baby.
Advanced Client Statement 3
[Hopeless] How can I possibly make challenging life decisions for myself? Every decision, big or small, was always made by my mother. Now, she's drunk all the time, or sick in bed, and I don't know what to do. I don't know how to take care of myself. I will never figure it out. It's too hard.
Advanced Client Statement 4
[Angry] I just don't know why you want me to express feelings. Feelings only lead to regrets and punishment. I was humiliated and punished when I showed any sign of sadness or fear to my father. He would always tell me that I would live to regret being such a weakling. I think he was right.
Advanced Client Statement 5
[Angry] I can't believe that you forgot the name of my neighbor who abused me! How could you forget?! Am I not important to you? Are you just like everyone else who pretends to listen but really ignores me? You say you care, but you're a liar. Everyone lies to me.

 Assess and adjust the difficulty here (see Step 3 in the exercise instructions). If appropriate, follow the instructions to make the exercise even more challenging (see Appendix A).

Example Therapist Responses: Limited Reparenting for the Angry and Vulnerable Child Modes

Remember: Trainees should attempt to improvise their own responses before reading the example responses. **Do not read the following responses verbatim unless you are having trouble coming up with your own responses!**

EXAMPLE RESPONSES TO BEGINNER-LEVEL CLIENT STATEMENTS FOR EXERCISE 9
Example Response to Beginner Client Statement 1
Of course it was extremely painful for you given the loneliness of your childhood. The vulnerable child part of you brings with her the feelings of despair from early times in your life. (Criterion 1) I want you to focus right now on our connection. Do you feel lonely here today with me? This is the place to start to give "little you" the connection she needs. (Criterion 2, Action 1)
Example Response to Beginner Client Statement 2
It is profoundly painful for anyone to feel that they don't matter to anyone. When you are in your vulnerable child mode all those painful feelings from childhood come back. (Criterion 1) Can you take in right now my saying that I see you and I would notice your absence if you disappeared? You matter to me. Try to let in the vulnerable part of you take this. (Criterion 2, Action 1)
Example Response to Beginner Client Statement 3
Of course you react when you feel like you are losing another person given the loss you experienced as a child. Your little vulnerable part is terrified when that happens. (Criterion 1) I don't feel tired of you, and I appreciate the courage it takes to express these fears. What would help you feel our connection right now? (Criterion 2, Action 1)
Example Response to Beginner Client Statement 4
It makes sense that your vulnerable part is expressing herself here as you remember the loss of your dad. Her hurts and her fears are understandable given that you had little support for emotional expression as a child. (Criterion 1) We need to be kind and patient with this part of you. Can we focus right now on our connection? This is a place to give "little you" the support she needs. (Criterion 2, Action 1)
Example Response to Beginner Client Statement 5
It must be so hard for that vulnerable part of you, when he senses that he is becoming the target of bullies again. As a child, he had no protection or safety, and he surely needed that. (Criterion 1) Let's see if we can bring some protection and comfort to this part of you now using safety imagery. Perhaps you might close your eyes and take a moment to see and sense him? I will guide you. (Criterion 2, Action 3)

EXAMPLE RESPONSES TO INTERMEDIATE-LEVEL CLIENT STATEMENTS FOR EXERCISE 9

Example Response to Intermediate Client Statement 1

Of course, you are angry. I get it. The little angry part of you feels the injustice you experienced deeply when he gets activated today. (Criterion 1) I am glad you are expressing it now. Let your angry child express it as much and as loud as you want. He is welcome here. (Criterion 2, Action 2)

Example Response to Intermediate Client Statement 2

I understand how hopeless it must feel when you recall your mother's neglect. Your vulnerable child feels the longing for secure connection and love that all kids need. (Criterion 1) I want us to look at how you could feel our connection securely now. What about moving your chair closer to mine so that you can feel my presence here with you and make more eye contact? How is this for you? (Criterion 2, Action 1)

Example Response to Intermediate Client Statement 3

Of course you wouldn't trust my words. It makes sense to me, as the vulnerable part of you had no one to count on, no one who showed any consistent caring and you could not safely express your anger as a little child. It will take time to have confidence in my caring. (Criterion 1) I welcome your expression of anger. Is there more anger you might want to express? (Criterion 2, Action 2)

Example Response to Intermediate Client Statement 4

I get it, that all of those panicky feelings are coming back when you consider being in a social situation. Your vulnerable child part imagines that she will experience that painful visibility of primary school. When this mode is triggered, you expect to be treated the same way you were back then. (Criterion 1) I suggest that you close your eyes and, using imagery, go back to your safe place. I will go with you so that you don't have to be alone there. (Criterion 2, Action 3)

Example Response to Intermediate Client Statement 5

Divorce is a painful experience for anyone, particularly because you had the experience of your dad leaving when you were little. Those memories and feelings all come back when your vulnerable child mode is triggered, like today. (Criterion 1) This is a safe place where you can share all these difficult feelings you've had to deal with for so long. (Criterion 2, Action 2)

EXAMPLE RESPONSES TO ADVANCED-LEVEL CLIENT STATEMENTS FOR EXERCISE 9

Example Response to Advanced Client Statement 1

Of course, that would be terrifying for anyone. It is bad enough for your adult self, but your vulnerable child part would feel the threat and that the danger was present, back to the time when she was not protected. (Criterion 1) Feel yourself here with me in my office where I will protect you and no one will be allowed to hurt you. Imagine the protective safety bubble around you and me that no one can break into. Whenever this memory comes up, use the bubble image for safety. (Criterion 2, Action 3)

Example Response to Advanced Client Statement 2

I am glad that you are expressing the anger you feel about this. It was not fair. Being ignored is a big trigger for you as your angry child mode remembers all the times your mother gave all her attention to your sister. You did not have the attention or time that every child needs to feel like they matter. (Criterion 1) Let yourself express all that you feel about this—give it voice. Only after you are able to do this will you know what action you really want to take today. (Criterion 2, Action 2)

Example Response to Advanced Client Statement 3

Of course, this feels really difficult for you as you have had no practice making these decisions. When you face an important decision, schemas get activated and then your anxious vulnerable child mode is triggered. No one taught you how to make decisions; they just did it for you. You needed guidance and support as a child so your confidence in your abilities would have grown. (Criterion 1) Fortunately, it is not too late to learn this, and I can help you learn to make decisions on your own. You're not alone. We will tackle this together. (Criterion 2, Action 1)

Example Response to Advanced Client Statement 4

I can understand how this doesn't make sense to you. The vulnerable part of you was shamed and threatened whenever you showed any feelings of distress to your father; you were made to feel as if you were being weak and that this could only lead to bad things for you in the future. (Criterion 1) But expressing your feelings is a natural way of communicating your needs as a child. All children need a safe place to express feelings. In fact, this can lead to positive outcomes in your life. I will help you experience this over time. (Criterion 2, Action 2)

Example Response to Advanced Client Statement 5

I understand how disappointed you are with me right now. My memory lapse set off your angry child mode, and you feel like you did with your dad as a child when he said he loved you but treated you as if you didn't matter. This part is really furious and tired of being treated this way. (Criterion 1) I am so sorry that I forgot the name. It is not because I don't care about you or that you are not important to me. It happened because I am not perfect and not good at remembering names. I understand too that it will take time and my caring behavior for you to trust that. I plan to hang in there with you until that happens. (Criterion 2, Action 1)

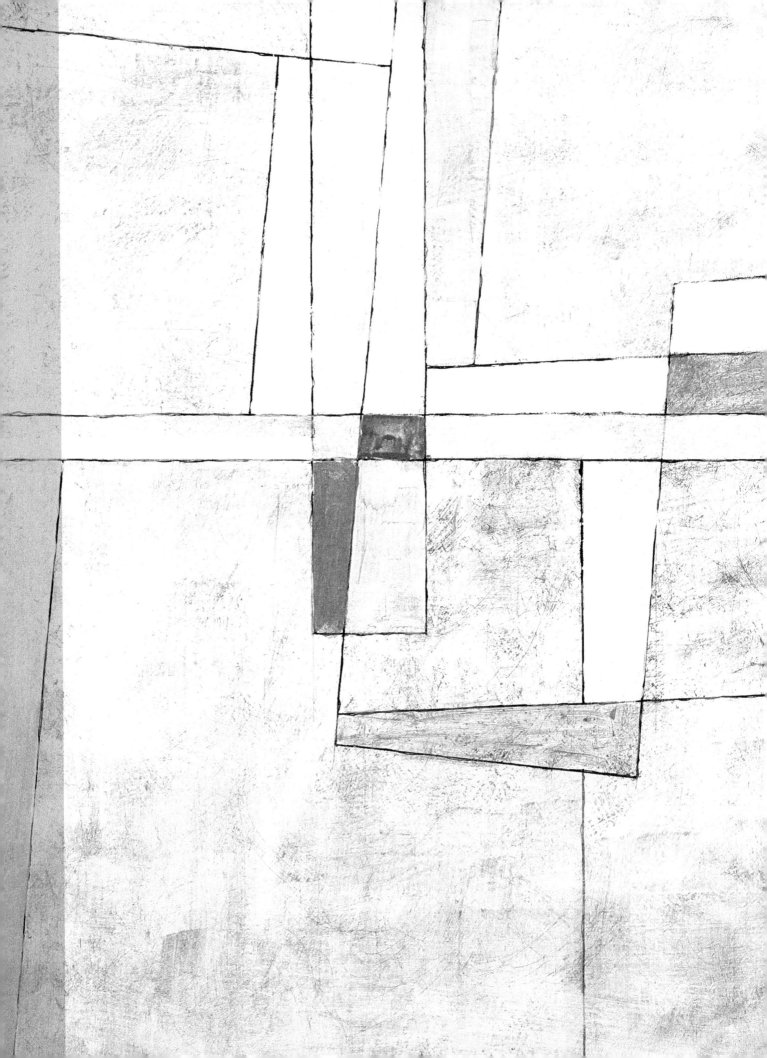

Limited Reparenting for the Demanding/Punitive Inner Critic Mode

Preparations for Exercise 10

1. Read the instructions in Chapter 2.

2. Download the Deliberate Practice Reaction Form and Deliberate Practice Diary Form at https://www.apa.org/pubs/books/deliberate-practice-schema-therapy (see the "Clinician and Practitioner Resources" tab; also available in Appendixes A and B, respectively).

Skill Description

Skill Difficulty Level: Advanced

This skill identifies and challenges the messages of the inner critic mode. The inner critic mode is typically the inherited/internalized critical, punitive, or demanding voice of a parent or other significant caregiver in the life of the child. Inner critic modes can also be derived from bullying or severe teasing during the client's childhood and adolescence. Under some circumstances, the inner critic may evolve from the mimicking of a parent or caregiver who modeled self-criticalness by launching demanding and harsh critical messages at themselves. The therapist aims to adapt, over time, the demanding and critical messages into caring and supportive ones, replacing the voice of the critic with the voice of a healthy, nurturing, and supportive "good parent."

For this exercise, the therapist improves a response to each client statement by first pointing out the presence of the inner critic mode and speculating about its childhood origins. The therapist continues by directly challenging this critic, labeling it as inaccurate, untrue, biased, unfair, or simply poorly delivered. Finally, the therapist provides a limited reparenting response by suggesting an alternative "good parent" message that

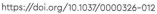

https://doi.org/10.1037/0000326-012

Deliberate Practice in Schema Therapy, by W. T. Behary, J. M. Farrell, A. Vaz, and T. Rousmaniere

meets a need present in the client's statement. This skill requires the therapist to act with a certain level of caring confidence to "stand up" convincingly to the critic mode and provide a supportive, corrective experience that counters the harsh messages the client may have received.

SKILL CRITERIA FOR EXERCISE 10

1. Point out the inner critic mode and speculate about its childhood origins.
2. Challenge the message of the critic as being inaccurate, untrue, biased, or unfair.
3. Suggest an alternative "good parent" message to meet the client's present need.

Examples of Limited Reparenting for the Demanding/Punitive Inner Critic Mode

Example 1

CLIENT: [*Sad*] I have been feeling lonely and sad since the divorce, but I know I am making a big deal of it and acting like a whiner, like always. I should just be able to close the chapter and get on with my life.

THERAPIST: Seems that you got the message, as a child, that your perfectly reasonable need to feel sad, to grieve, or to hurt was labeled as "whiny" or "weak," which led to this internal critic that now shows up when there is hurt. (Criterion 1) Loss is very hard, no matter what the circumstances might be. It's not fair that this critic part is being so hard on you. (Criterion 2) It's important that we acknowledge the sadness and make room for the grief and pain of your loss. You are just sad, and it makes sense. You are entitled to those feelings. (Criterion 3)

Example 2

CLIENT: [*Hopeless*] I don't know why I expected the date to go well. I should just accept that I am a loser who no one wants to be around. Even my mother didn't particularly like me and said I was a disappointment.

THERAPIST: Your mother clearly had some issues, leaving you feeling like you were not worthy of anyone's attention. It's no wonder you developed this internal critic mode which is so tough on you. You still feel that harsh message right in your bones. (Criterion 1) Despite whatever your mother's intentions might have been, she was wrong to say such things to an innocent little child. (Criterion 2) It's painful to experience the feeling of being rejected or ignored. But I think you and I could find a reasonable way to understand what actually happened on that date and help you with these feelings. (Criterion 3)

Example 3

CLIENT: [*Anxious*] I am so afraid that I will also drive you away, just like everyone else in my life. You must be so fed up with me. All I do is whine about my life. I don't do anything about it. I am sick of myself.

THERAPIST: This is your inner critic mode, the part that is impatient, harsh, and demanding. You probably heard some of these critical messages in your past, in one form or another, and they stuck around. (Criterion 1) These critical messages are really unfair and unhelpful to you. (Criterion 2) I care very much about you. It's scary facing new challenges. You have shown so much courage just letting me get to know you, and it's a privilege to know you. I think you might need to try out a new message, such as, "I am fine as I am, and I will continue to grow, learn, and make healthy choices, in my own time and in my own way." And to your inner critic you might say, "Just, leave me alone!" (Criterion 3)

INSTRUCTIONS FOR EXERCISE 10
Step 1: Role-Play and Feedback
• The client says the first beginner client statement. The therapist improvises a response based on the skill criteria. • The trainer (or, if not available, the client) provides brief feedback based on the skill criteria. • The client then repeats the same statement, and the therapist again improvises a response. The trainer (or client) again provides brief feedback.
Step 2: Repeat
• Repeat Step 1 for all the statements in the current difficulty level (beginner, intermediate, or advanced).
Step 3: Assess and Adjust Difficulty
• The therapist completes the Deliberate Practice Reaction Form (see Appendix A) and decides whether to make the exercise easier or harder or to repeat the same difficulty level.
Step 4: Repeat for Approximately 15 Minutes
• Repeat Steps 1 to 3 for at least 15 minutes. • The trainees then switch therapist and client roles and start over.

> **Now it's your turn! Follow Steps 1 and 2 from the instructions.**

Remember: The goal of the role-play is for trainees to practice improvising responses to the client statements in a manner that (a) uses the skill criteria and (b) feels authentic for the trainee. **Example therapist responses for each client statement are provided at the end of this exercise. Trainees should attempt to improvise their own responses before reading the example responses.**

BEGINNER-LEVEL CLIENT STATEMENTS FOR EXERCISE 10
Beginner Client Statement 1
[Sad] You are very nice and caring to me, but that's because you're a therapist. That's what you are supposed to do. **[Disgusted]** I can't imagine how anyone in the real world would want to put up with me if they really knew me. I learned long ago that I am just a pathetic loser. It's not surprising that my phone never rings and I am never invited to any social events.
Beginner Client Statement 2
[Fearful] I don't know how I am ever going to give this presentation in front of the committee. **[Agitated]** I have prepared and prepared for months, but I know it's not enough. I will never be as interesting or entertaining as my colleagues when they make a presentation. My father was right. The best I can ever expect is that I will make a fool of myself if I let others see the real me.
Beginner Client Statement 3
[Sad] I was so hoping that maybe he would ask me to join him for dinner. I thought we were making a good connection. What an idiot I am! What was I thinking? I can hear my mother's warning in my brain. I am just so ugly and boring. Why would a good-looking, charming, and intelligent guy like that want to date someone like me?
Beginner Client Statement 4
[Exasperated] I'm sorry. I know you are doing your best to help me. It must be so frustrating for you having to deal with someone like me. It's the story of my life, always has been. I don't follow through on anything. All I do is complain, I am destined to be stuck in an unhappy life, and it's all my fault. I really cannot stand myself anymore!
Beginner Client Statement 5
[Sad] I have been feeling lonely and sad since the divorce, but I know I am making a big deal of it and acting like a whiner. I should just be able to close the chapter and get on with my life.

 Assess and adjust the difficulty before moving to the next difficulty level (see Step 3 in the exercise instructions).

INTERMEDIATE-LEVEL CLIENT STATEMENTS FOR EXERCISE 10

Intermediate Client Statement 1

[Worried] I can't believe I was given a promotion at work. I am such a fraud. They just don't know how terribly lazy and stupid I am and how much time I spend doing work at home in the evening and on weekends, just to keep up with my deadlines. Soon they will discover what my parents always knew—that I am incompetent. They will probably take away the promotion. It's gonna be so embarrassing.

Intermediate Client Statement 2

[Hopeless] I don't know why I expected the date to go well. I should just accept that I am a loser who no one wants to be around. Even my mother didn't particularly like me and said I was a disappointment.

Intermediate Client Statement 3

[Anxious] I am so afraid that I will also drive you away, just like everyone else in my life. You must be so fed up with me. I know I have made some progress, but I don't try hard enough. I am constantly avoiding everything that makes me uncomfortable. All I do is whine about my life. I don't do anything about it. I am sick of myself.

Intermediate Client Statement 4

[Angry] I feel very angry right now, and I have no right to feel this way. I am the one who destroys my friendships. I push people away. I am too sensitive and demanding and needy. I cry too easily and expect everyone to feel sorry for me—how pathetic! My mother was right. I am damaged goods.

Intermediate Client Statement 5

[Hopeless] Why can I never get it right? I lost another sale this week, and my boss was clearly disappointed. I can't blame him. I am not working hard enough. I know my associate would have done a much better job securing this sale. I am not clever enough. This is just like having to compete with my big brother. My dad always said he would be a success and I would end up living in a box.

 Assess and adjust the difficulty before moving to the next difficulty level (see Step 3 in the exercise instructions).

ADVANCED-LEVEL CLIENT STATEMENTS FOR EXERCISE 10

Advanced Client Statement 1

[Angry] You probably don't believe me, but I was really looking forward to this session. If I was smart enough, I would have left my house a little early to avoid the traffic. But I am so stupid, and I didn't pay attention to the time again, and now I'm late. I yelled at myself the whole way here. I am tired of being me.

Advanced Client Statement 2

[Sad] I don't deserve to be happy. It's my fault that my mother is lonely all the time. I don't call her enough; I don't show enough gratitude for all that she has given me. I am selfish. I should be living with her and keeping her company. I mean, I don't have a life anyway. If something happens to her, she says I will live to regret my actions. She is probably right about that too.

Advanced Client Statement 3

[Hopeless] I am just not good enough. I failed one part of my licensing exam again and will have to take it over. I just don't have what it takes to be a doctor. My father told me I should not try to take on such a difficult job—that it was beyond me.

Advanced Client Statement 4

[Regretful] I have spent so many years in therapy. What is wrong with me? How could it take so long to realize that I was living in a destructive relationship? Why didn't I see it sooner? Maybe I liked being mistreated. Perhaps I am just a drama queen looking for attention. My mother was right. What a waste of time. I will never forgive myself.

Advanced Client Statement 5

[Frightened] I got as far as the parking lot, and I froze. I couldn't get myself to walk into the restaurant. When am I going to grow up and get over this ridiculous phobia? I am a 45-year-old woman and I act like a weak little pathetic child who is afraid of ghosts. I am an embarrassment.

 Assess and adjust the difficulty here (see Step 3 in the exercise instructions). If appropriate, follow the instructions to make the exercise even more challenging (see Appendix A).

Example Therapist Responses: Limited Reparenting for the Demanding/Punitive Inner Critic Mode

Remember: Trainees should attempt to improvise their own responses before reading the example responses. **Do not read the following responses verbatim unless you are having trouble coming up with your own responses!**

EXAMPLE RESPONSES TO BEGINNER-LEVEL CLIENT STATEMENTS FOR EXERCISE 10
Example Response to Beginner Client Statement 1
This sounds like your internal critic mode getting triggered. That's the part of you that becomes unfairly harsh and shaming toward you. When you were just a child, you were made to feel that you were not worthy of love and attention. (Criterion 1) This message was not only hurtful, it was also wrong. (Criterion 2) Every child, including you, deserves to be loved and attended to. I am caring toward you because you are worthy of that care. You are a good person, and I am going to help you to make those important and meaningful connections that are missing in your life. (Criterion 3)
Example Response to Beginner Client Statement 2
I am detecting the voice of your internal critic mode—the voice of your father who could never see the goodness and beauty in his precious child. (Criterion 1) Nothing is ever good enough for this critic, and he always predicts a bad outcome. And he must be silenced because despite whatever protection he was trying to promote, he hurt you with this false message. (Criterion 2) No one is perfect, but we are all good enough in our own way. You have prepared well, and you don't need to be perfect. You just need to be you. That's good enough. (Criterion 3)
Example Response to Beginner Client Statement 3
Every child needs to feel cherished and accepted by their caregivers. This sounds like the internal critic showing up now, your mother's voice just as you noticed. (Criterion 1) The message is harsh and terribly unfair, and it's also not true. (Criterion 2) You are a lovely person, and surely there's another reason why John didn't invite you. I will help you consider the alternatives as we work together to silence this inner critic mode. (Criterion 3)
Example Response to Beginner Client Statement 4
This sounds like your internal critic mode speaking right now. It's distressing to hear how harsh it can be when you are struggling. There was never anyone to guide and support you when you were little, as every child needs. (Criterion 1) Your inner critic immediately puts you down and is punitive when you aren't perfect, and this must stop. We must be allies in fighting these false messages together. (Criterion 2) I see someone in front of me who has struggled and is working hard to heal and make difficult choices. The process is slow, but she is good, and she is growing. (Criterion 3)
Example Response to Beginner Client Statement 5
Seems you got the message, as a child, that your perfectly reasonable need to feel sad, to grieve, or to hurt was labeled as "whiny" or "weak," which led to this internal critic that shows up when you feel hurt. (Criterion 1) Loss is very hard, no matter what the circumstances might be. It's not fair that this critic part is being so harsh. It's important that we acknowledge the sadness and make room for the grief and pain of your loss. (Criterion 2) You are just sad, and it makes sense. You are entitled to those feelings. (Criterion 3)

EXAMPLE RESPONSES TO INTERMEDIATE-LEVEL CLIENT STATEMENTS FOR EXERCISE 10

Example Response to Intermediate Client Statement 1

How sad that you were taught that you cannot trust your own capacities. Every child needs to be praised and recognized for their efforts and supported in their struggles. This is clearly your inner critic mode getting activated, based on your parents' early messages. (Criterion 1) Those negative statements are unjustified. And even though this critic may be trying to prevent you from the surprise of some embarrassing outcome, the delivery is inaccurate, harsh, and unacceptable. (Criterion 2) You earned this promotion because you work extra hard—even more than is fair to yourself. You are doing fine, and you are entitled to celebrate this victory. (Criterion 3)

Example Response to Intermediate Client Statement 2

Your mother clearly had some issues, leaving you feeling like you were not worthy of anyone's attention. It's no wonder you developed this internal critic mode that is so tough on you. You still feel that harsh message right in your bones. (Criterion 1) Despite whatever your mother's intentions might have been, she was wrong to say such things to a precious and innocent little child. (Criterion 2) It's painful to experience the feeling of being rejected or ignored. But I think you and I could find a reasonable way to understand what actually happened on that date and help you with these feelings. (Criterion 3)

Example Response to Intermediate Client Statement 3

This is your inner critic mode, the part that's impatient, harsh, and demanding. You probably heard some of these critical messages in your past, in one form or another, and they stuck around. (Criterion 1) At the end of the day, these critical messages are really unfair and unhelpful to you. (Criterion 2) I care very much about you. It's scary facing new challenges. You have shown so much courage just letting me get to know you, and it's a privilege to know you. I think you might need to try out a new message, such as, "I am fine as I am, and I will continue to grow, learn, and make healthy choices, in my own time and in my own way." And to your inner critic you might say, "Just leave me alone!" (Criterion 3)

Example Response to Intermediate Client Statement 4

This is your critic mode speaking now. It's the internal message coming from your mother, who was unable to meet your normal need for love and attention when you were a child. (Criterion 1) Instead, she just blamed you by calling you "damaged goods," which was punitive and unacceptable. No child is damaged goods. (Criterion 2) You were like every other child who is naturally needy, sensitive, loveable, and innocent, and we can look more carefully at what's happening in your friendships without the harsh blame and criticalness that only hurts you. (Criterion 3)

Example Response to Intermediate Client Statement 5

You learned that you would never get it right from your dad, from the time you were very young. This is your inner critic mode, and when things are not perfect, it gets activated, becoming harsh and hurtful to you. (Criterion 1) How unfair that your dad would compare you to your older brother and not value you for being you, forcing you to compete in ways that were unreasonable. It's not okay, it was never okay. (Criterion 2) We are all entitled to have a bad day or go through a bad phase in our work. We cannot always get it right. You're fine and you don't need to compete for your father's approval. We will figure this out together. (Criterion 3)

EXAMPLE RESPONSES TO ADVANCED-LEVEL CLIENT STATEMENTS FOR EXERCISE 10

Example Response to Advanced Client Statement 1

All children need guidance and support, praise, and acceptance from the grownups they depend on. This sounds like an inner critic mode that has developed from your grandfather's unrealistic expectations of you, filled with harsh messages. (Criterion 1) It is way too extreme to call yourself stupid. Your grandfather was wrong, expecting too much and overreacting. (Criterion 2) You cannot always know how busy the traffic will be. You are not stupid when you make a mistake or you face an obstacle. That's just how life happens sometimes. Of course I believe you wanted to be here, and I am so happy that you made it despite the traffic. (Criterion 3)

Example Response to Advanced Client Statement 2

Wow, those messages don't leave any room for you to be happy as if you were brought into this world only to take care of your mother. This sounds like a very strong inner critic mode has been activated. (Criterion 1) A mother's role is to love and protect her child, to encourage her child, to grow and discover their identity. It was her job to support your autonomy. It was not you who was self-absorbed. (Criterion 2) You deserve to be happy. You have been so devoted to your mom even when it meant giving up your own rights and needs. You are so caring, and you have the right to have a life of your own. (Criterion 3)

Example Response to Advanced Client Statement 3

This is your critic mode getting activated right in this moment. And you immediately get reminded of the messages coming from your father. Sounds like he taught you how to lose confidence in yourself if you make a mistake, to avoid challenges. (Criterion 1) You failed only one part of the exam, but that's all your critic focuses on, and that isn't fair. It does not mean that you cannot be a doctor. Your father's evaluation was unfair and overly negative, and now your critic is echoing him. This is not acceptable. (Criterion 2) You are good enough, but sometimes we all face challenges, and we can try again if we choose to. You can opt to take the exam again. (Criterion 3)

Example Response to Advanced Client Statement 4

Wow! I hear your critic loud and clear in those messages! All children need the grownups in their lives to provide comfort and attention when they are upset. (Criterion 1) Your mother was unable to meet your natural needs and instead gave you a very biased message about yourself—one that is completely false and unfair. (Criterion 2) No one likes to be mistreated, and you didn't like it either. Not from your mother and now not from your partner. You are understanding things more clearly now, you are healing. Relationships can be very complicated. You are fine. (Criterion 3)

Example Response to Advanced Client Statement 5

All children have times of being fearful and need their caretakers to comfort them and help them feel secure. This is clearly an inner critic mode getting activated, sending harshly critical messages to you at a time when you were scared. (Criterion 1) How sad and unfair for anyone to give a 5-year-old child such a message when she is feeling afraid. She needs soothing comfort and a voice of gentle encouragement, not judgment and meanness. (Criterion 2) I will help you create accurate messages for the little child in you, as well as for your grown-up self. You made it to the parking lot this time. That was a big step for you. We make progress in steps, and I am proud of you. (Criterion 3)

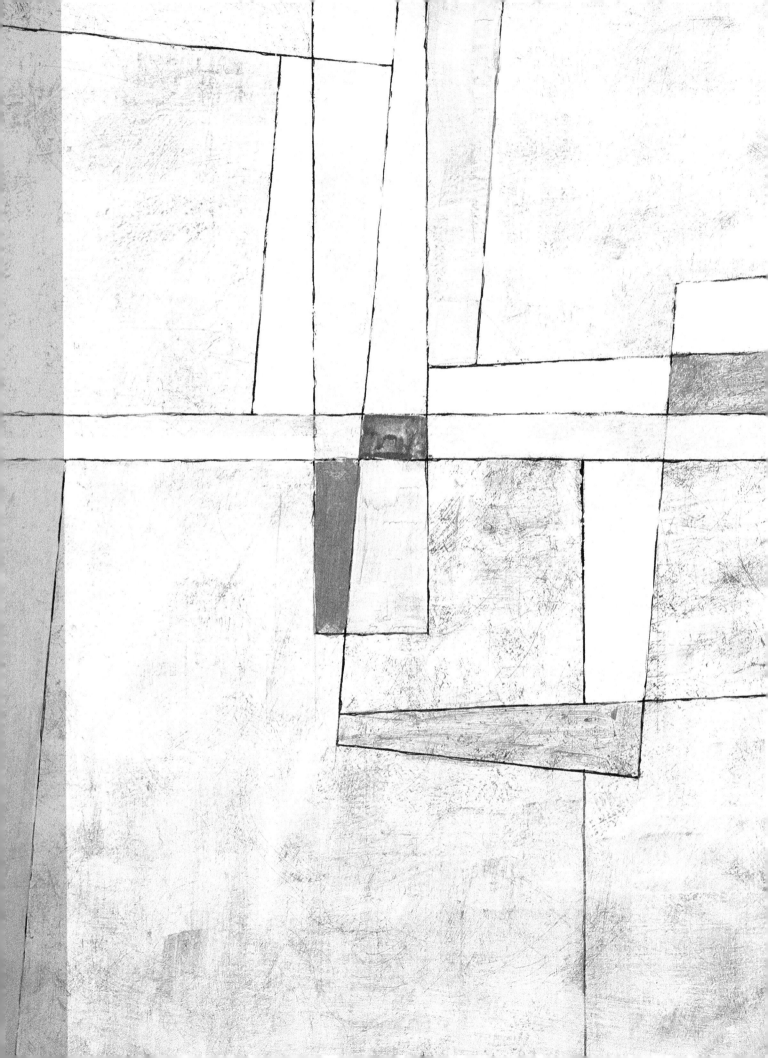

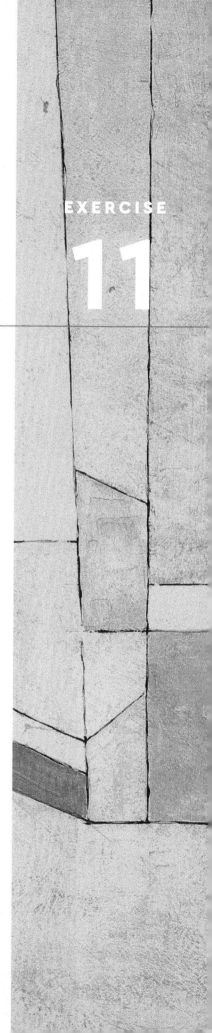

Limited Reparenting for the Maladaptive Coping Modes: Empathic Confrontation

Preparations for Exercise 11

1. Read the instructions in Chapter 2.

2. Download the Deliberate Practice Reaction Form and Deliberate Practice Diary Form at https://www.apa.org/pubs/books/deliberate-practice-schema-therapy (see the "Clinician and Practitioner Resources" tab; also available in Appendixes A and B, respectively).

Skill Description

Skill Difficulty Level: Advanced

Empathic confrontation is a limited reparenting response used to address maladaptive coping modes. The therapist points out the problematic behaviors showing up in the coping mode in terms of how they do not meet the client's needs. For example, pushing people away with bully–attack behaviors prevents the connection the client needs in close relationships. The therapist's empathy is used to express a clear understanding of the reasons for these coping mode behaviors, based on early experience and constructed patterns (modes) for coping, while also pointing out how these patterns are self-defeating and block getting the client's needs met. It is critical to confront the targeted behavior when it prevents clients' healthy interpersonal and practical functioning because this is a key component of personality disorder issues.

For this exercise, the therapist first highlights the client's problematic coping mode behavior and its consequences, using a warm, noncritical tone. Although each client statement notes which maladaptive coping mode the client is expressing (e.g., avoidant protector mode; see also Appendix C for a list of the coping modes), the therapist does not need to identify the specific coping mode present in their response. The therapist then empathically communicates that this behavioral pattern is a leftover

https://doi.org/10.1037/0000326-013

Deliberate Practice in Schema Therapy, by W. T. Behary, J. M. Farrell, A. Vaz, and T. Rousmaniere

survival response from childhood. Finally, the therapist suggests a specific alternative behavior that is more likely to help the client in meeting their needs. Overall, these interventions convey that clients are not at fault for having developed problematic patterns, are worthy of their needs, and are capable of finding new, more adaptive ways to meet them.

SKILL CRITERIA FOR EXERCISE 11
1. Point out in a warm, noncritical way how a coping mode behavior is problematic because it does not get the client's need met.
2. Communicate the understanding that this is a leftover survival response from childhood when a core need was not met.
3. Suggest that an alternative behavior is necessary to get the client's need met.

Examples of Limited Reparenting for the Maladaptive Coping Modes: Empathic Confrontation

Example 1

CLIENT: [*Annoyed, avoidant protector mode*] I just don't feel things. I am more of a thinker, less emotional. I also don't see the value in bringing up emotions. My wife keeps complaining that I never tell her how I feel. It's just painful and it doesn't lead to anything anyway. If I had reacted to all of the emotions I felt growing up in my crazy, dysfunctional family, I wouldn't have survived. Like my dad liked to say, "Talk to the hand."

THERAPIST: I understand that when "the wall" goes up, it blocks out all emotions, but it also interferes with you getting your needs met. This is part of the reason why you are struggling in your personal relationships. (Criterion 1) It's not your fault, it's what you learned. You developed this mode to protect yourself in a very chaotic and demanding childhood environment. Emotions were not tolerated, and you were made to feel weak and ashamed when you expressed them as a little child. (Criterion 2) We can unlearn these biased emotional messages so that you can have the deep and meaningful connections that you need—that you always needed. (Criterion 3)

Example 2

CLIENT: [*Ashamed, compliant surrender to self-sacrifice mode*] I know I called you twice last week and I'm so sorry. I should have been able to handle that situation on my own. I know you have a busy life and are entitled to a break from your clients. I learned about how much I could do on my own at home growing up. There were bigger things going on than little me with my mom drinking and my dad always in a rage. I am doing fine now. I brought you some flowers to thank you. I actually don't have much to talk about today. How was your week?

THERAPIST: That is very thoughtful of you. I appreciate your kindness. However, I think it reflects your coping mode, which has you always concerned about the other person's needs and never your own. It keeps you voiceless and frustrated in your adult relationships as your needs are never met. (Criterion 1) I suspect you might have learned to cope this way a long time ago, giving in to demands and sacrificing your needs and opinions, especially when your home was scary, with your mom drinking and your dad raging.

(Criterion 2) I am glad you called me during that crisis, and I was happy to be able to help you. You are not a burden to me. You don't have to sacrifice your needs with me. I am here for you. This is your space. (Criterion 3)

Example 3

CLIENT: [*Angry, self-aggrandizer mode*] I don't see why I shouldn't get a full session. There was a lot of traffic, and I had a board meeting that caused me to be late for the session. This is ridiculous. You just don't understand how important my job is. My dad taught me that super-achievers are the people who count. They get different rules and special privileges. I am the president of my company. But I wouldn't expect you to understand this since you're only a therapist.

THERAPIST: I cannot give you the extra time because it wouldn't be fair to my other clients or to me. Your expectation that you should have special rules is part of the reason you are having problems in your relationships with coworkers—and in your marriage too. (Criterion 1) I understand that your dad taught you that you will be able to do and have whatever you want, without consequence, as if you were entitled to special privileges and special rules. (Criterion 2) This is not your fault, but it is definitely something you need to change if you want your marriage and other relationships to work. Relationships are about give-and-take, limits, and consequences. (Criterion 3)

INSTRUCTIONS FOR EXERCISE 11

Step 1: Role-Play and Feedback

- The client says the first beginner client statement. The therapist improvises a response based on the skill criteria.
- The trainer (or, if not available, the client) provides brief feedback based on the skill criteria.
- The client then repeats the same statement, and the therapist again improvises a response. The trainer (or client) again provides brief feedback.

Step 2: Repeat

- Repeat Step 1 for all the statements in the current difficulty level (beginner, intermediate, or advanced).

Step 3: Assess and Adjust Difficulty

- The therapist completes the Deliberate Practice Reaction Form (see Appendix A) and decides whether to make the exercise easier or harder or to repeat the same difficulty level.

Step 4: Repeat for Approximately 15 Minutes

- Repeat Steps 1 to 3 for at least 15 minutes.
- The trainees then switch therapist and client roles and start over.

> **Now it's your turn! Follow Steps 1 and 2 from the instructions.**

Remember: The goal of the role-play is for trainees to practice improvising responses to the client statements in a manner that (a) uses the skill criteria and (b) feels authentic for the trainee. **Example therapist responses for each client statement are provided at the end of this exercise. Trainees should attempt to improvise their own responses before reading the example responses.**

BEGINNER-LEVEL CLIENT STATEMENTS FOR EXERCISE 11
Beginner Client Statement 1
[Sad, avoidant protector mode] I felt really sad and shed a few tears when my friend called last-minute and canceled our plans. **[Upbeat tone]** I don't know why I am reacting so much; it is really not a big deal at all.
Beginner Client Statement 2
[Angry, angry protector mode] I was cheated by not having the opportunity to really know my father. I didn't really miss anything—he was a jerk.
Beginner Client Statement 3
[Sad, detached protector mode] I never felt loved as a child or that I mattered to anyone. **[Disoriented]** Is that what you asked me about? My mind just went blank.
Beginner Client Statement 4
[Sad, self-aggrandizer mode] Once again, no one invited me to lunch today. My coworkers make their lunch plans and overlook me like I am invisible. You know what? Who needs them! They are all boring and not very interesting anyway. They're just jealous of me.
Beginner Client Statement 5
[Angry, detached protector mode] I feel angry right now when I think about how little safety I had as a child. It was criminal the way I was treated. But I think I am being too sensitive. What doesn't kill you makes you stronger.

 Assess and adjust the difficulty before moving to the next difficulty level (see Step 3 in the exercise instructions).

INTERMEDIATE-LEVEL CLIENT STATEMENTS FOR EXERCISE 11

Intermediate Client Statement 1

[Anxious, compliant surrender to self-sacrifice mode] I should have cancelled my session today as I needed the time to finish the prep for my boss's presentation tomorrow. It is an important one for her and even staying up all night and skipping meals has not given me enough time to do the job she needs from me. As a child, my mother was very ill, and we all had to focus on taking care of her. There was often little sleep or even meals, but it was a life-or-death situation. Maybe I can leave early today after 20 minutes so I can get back to work?

Intermediate Client Statement 2

[Flat, compliant surrender to abandonment mode] Everyone leaves me. You will be no exception. You cannot count on anyone. It has always been that way. My father died before I was born, and my mother committed suicide when I was 6 months old. Why would I think anything else was possible for me? So I never married, and I use relationships for casual sex—no commitment.

Intermediate Client Statement 3

[Anxious, compliant surrender to subjugation mode] I get so scared when I disagree with my wife even about small things. I feel like I did with my father as a child. If I said anything he did not like he started to yell and sometimes even hit me. It just wasn't worth the risk with him, and it feels the same now. The problem is that we never do things my way unless she suggests it.

Intermediate Client Statement 4

[Sad, compliant surrender to self-sacrifice mode] The death of my grandma has been one of the most difficult losses I've ever experienced. She was the only person who really loved me just for me while everyone else was busy placing enormous guilt on me anytime I showed any emotions at all. But there are more important things to focus on now. I should be thinking about how to help my little brother to prepare for his upcoming job interview. I think there will be a lot of applicants for this position and the competition will be hard for him.

Intermediate Client Statement 5

[Anxious, compliant surrender to self-sacrifice mode] I am worried about not having enough time today to address all of the conflict that I am dealing with this week. And I know I shouldn't be asking for extra time from you. I mean I know you care, and you give a lot, and I don't want you to think I am not appreciative of you. I really am. And even as I say this, I can hear my mother telling me to stop being so selfish. I'm so sorry. I can only imagine that I have offended you by seeming so ungrateful and so needy.

 Assess and adjust the difficulty before moving to the next difficulty level (see Step 3 in the exercise instructions).

ADVANCED-LEVEL CLIENT STATEMENTS FOR EXERCISE 11
Advanced Client Statement 1
[Angry, self-aggrandizing mode] I don't see why I shouldn't get a full session. There was a lot of traffic, and I had an important meeting that caused me to be late for the session. This is ridiculous. You just don't understand how important my job is. I am the president of my company. But I wouldn't expect you to understand this since you are only a therapist. You probably never learned that when you work hard and you are extremely successful, you have the right to special privileges.
Advanced Client Statement 2
[Frustrated, angry protector mode] Well, this is the way it's always been for me. My brother and sister were allowed to be actual children, to make mistakes, to play, to be afraid of things. Not me. I was "chosen" to be the tough guy, the brave one, the perfect one. This is ridiculous. Why are you asking me all these stupid questions? It's all in the past and you cannot change it. You're just like my partner, always looking for "feelings." Feelings are a waste of time. They don't pay the bills.
Advanced Client Statement 3
[Frustrated, bully–attack mode] Yes, I am still having trouble with sleep, and I am having trouble getting along at work. I am sad about losing my marriage, but I don't know why I have to talk about how I felt when my ex left me. That was long ago, and I don't see what it has to do with anything now. You are starting to sound like a second-rate television psychologist. I could hear my dad if he knew I was talking to you. He would be laughing at me saying that nothing good comes from self-pity; therapists just want to make you cry so they can feel successful.
Advanced Client Statement 4
[Upbeat, self-aggrandizing mode] Yeah, we can talk about my relationship issues later. I assume you're wondering about my weekend. Well, not only did I purchase the most fabulous and expensive suit for the event, but I was seated next to the most famous professor. I know this was intentional because the chairperson of the event knows of my success with the university and all my very generous donations to the department. I don't mean to brag, but I thought you would find it interesting. I know my mom would find this very entertaining if she were alive. This is really all that mattered to her when it came to her children. Make her look good no matter what!
Advanced Client Statement 5
[Suspicious and angry, bully–attack mode] So, you say you care about me and my family. But, let's face it, this is a business transaction. I pay you and you say nice things to me. That's really all it is. I learned a long time ago that when people say nice things to you, they just want something from you. My mom could be very sweet when she wanted me to make her look good in front of her friends. I was the trophy for her. I trust no one but myself. Don't take this the wrong way, but I am smarter than most people anyway. I studied psychology too.

 Assess and adjust the difficulty here (see Step 3 in the exercise instructions). If appropriate, follow the instructions to make the exercise even more challenging (see Appendix A).

Example Therapist Responses: Limited Reparenting for the Maladaptive Coping Modes: Empathic Confrontation

Remember: Trainees should attempt to improvise their own responses before reading the example responses. **Do not read the following responses verbatim unless you are having trouble coming up with your own responses!**

EXAMPLE RESPONSES TO BEGINNER-LEVEL CLIENT STATEMENTS FOR EXERCISE 11
Example Response to Beginner Client Statement 1
When you feel something painful, like sadness and then quickly question your feelings and minimize them, you are cutting off important information about what you need. (Criterion 1) I know this is a coping response from childhood when your feelings were criticized or minimized. (Criterion 2) But you need to take your sadness seriously and explore what it communicates to you about what you need. (Criterion 3)
Example Response to Beginner Client Statement 2
Your anger is legitimate and gives you important information about a basic need that was not met for you in childhood. When you dismiss it today, you may deny your need for connection. (Criterion 1) You could not do anything as a child to change your dad's availability, so you had to push down your anger about it. (Criterion 2) Today you need to be aware of your feelings in relationships to know whether that person is available and your need for healthy connection can be met with them. (Criterion 3)
Example Response to Beginner Client Statement 3
I think that you detached just now because feeling unloved and unimportant is so painful, but then you are just left with emptiness and numbness. (Criterion 1) Your survival as a child in an environment without love or care depended on not feeling that overwhelming pain. (Criterion 2) Today there are actions you can take to get the love and attention you deserve if you can stay present and don't numb out emotionally or disappear. (Criterion 3)
Example Response to Beginner Client Statement 4
You started to feel the safety of our connection then felt the anxiety of taking that risk and cut it off. (Criterion 1) As a child, you had no reliable, supportive adult to count on, so it's understandable that you fear and avoid relying on anyone. (Criterion 2) However, you need connection now and did so back then as well. Our relationship can be a safe place to take the risk of relying on our relationship. (Criterion 3)
Example Response to Beginner Client Statement 5
Of course you feel angry! All children need and deserve safety. Hang onto your anger so that the "good parent" part of you never compromises on the safety "little you" needs. (Criterion 1) Your lack of safety as a child might have killed you if you hadn't found ways to detach from it. (Criterion 2) Today you need to be aware of this anger when you are in unsafe situations so that you do not take risks with your safety and put yourself in harm's way. (Criterion 3)

EXAMPLE RESPONSES TO INTERMEDIATE-LEVEL CLIENT STATEMENTS FOR EXERCISE 11

Example Response to Intermediate Client Statement 1

Wow, your devotion to your boss's needs sounds limitless. What about you? You need these therapy sessions, and you certainly need sleep and nourishment. (Criterion 1) You grew up in an environment where your mother's needs were huge and always came first in the family. There was very little left over for you and you learned to deny your needs and just get by. (Criterion 2) However, your needs are just as important today as they were when you were a child, and today they should not always be put aside for someone else's. (Criterion 3)

Example Response to Intermediate Client Statement 2

I am so sad thinking of "little you" having no one and accepting that no one will ever stay—not even your therapist—and you will always be alone. (Criterion 1) It's no wonder you have that message given your tragic history, (Criterion 2) but when you act as if your belief that no one will ever stay is truth, it keeps you from taking the emotional risks involved in connecting, which are required to develop the important relationships you want and we all need. (Criterion 3)

Example Response to Intermediate Client Statement 3

So your need to be autonomous or part of the decision making in your family is never met and your wife may not even be aware of this. (Criterion 1) It is understandable that your childhood experience of fear and even punishment for having your own wants or needs led to keeping quiet. (Criterion 2) However, today as an adult, you have a right to be heard regarding what you want and need and to be an equal in decision making. This will only happen if you can overcome the old messages and take a chance in relationships that feel safer. (Criterion 3)

Example Response to Intermediate Client Statement 4

I notice that as soon as you begin to feel your sadness while reflecting on the painful loss of your grandma—the one person who loved you unconditionally—you switch into that part of you that causes you to feel guilty when you focus on yourself and your needs. (Criterion 1) Of course, you feel the need to focus on your brother, given all the guilt that was placed upon you. It was only your grandma who allowed you to express your feelings. (Criterion 2) But every time you depart from your feelings, that vulnerable part of you gets neglected again, made to feel guilty, and your needs don't get met. And in this space with me, your feelings and needs matter. I would like to hear more about your sadness. You are entitled to feel your grief. (Criterion 3)

Example Response to Intermediate Client Statement 5

There is a part of you that is really struggling to ask for my help and the need for some extra time. At the same time, another part of you starts to apologize as you imagine that you've offended me. (Criterion 1) I can imagine that giving in to the voice of your mother might help you to feel less guilt and selfishness, but it also blocks your opportunity to ask for the support you need and the care you deserve. (Criterion 2) You always needed and deserved this care, and you are never a burden to me. In fact, I am very proud of you for having the courage to ask for the extra time. You advocated for yourself and did not offend me. (Criterion 3)

EXAMPLE RESPONSES TO ADVANCED-LEVEL CLIENT STATEMENTS FOR EXERCISE 11

Example Response to Advanced Client Statement 1

I cannot give you the extra time because it wouldn't be fair to my other clients or to me. Your expectation that you should have special rules is part of the reason you are having problems in your relationships with coworkers—and in your marriage too. (Criterion 1) I understand that growing up with a dad who told you that all you have to do is be an extraordinary achiever and you will be able to do and have whatever you want, without consequence, no limits made you feel as if you were entitled to special privileges and special rules. (Criterion 2) This is not your fault, but it is definitely something you need to change if you want your marriage and other relationships to work. Relationships are about give-and-take, limits, and consequences. (Criterion 3)

Example Response to Advanced Client Statement 2

There's that part of you again that keeps me from feeling closer to you by becoming critical of the therapy, and of our connection. (Criterion 1) This is not your fault; this is what you were taught. You were expected to stop being a little child and to meet unrealistic demands, but it is your responsibility, with my help, to confront this message and to allow your feelings to be felt and shared. (Criterion 2) This is an unmet need and part of the reason your partner is hurting and your relationship is suffering. I can help you with this, but we will have to ask this tough guy part to step aside. (Criterion 3)

Example Response to Advanced Client Statement 3

There's that tough part of you. The part that shuts down all connection to reasonable sadness and becomes suspicious and critical of therapy and the therapist's motivations. (Criterion 1) It's clear that your father had you believe that you are wasting time when you allow yourself to experience difficult emotions, and that you should not trust anyone who wants to know you in this deep and personal way. But this is why you are still struggling with sleep and getting along with coworkers. The sadness of the breakup is valid and painful and needs a space to be felt and grieved, just like all the feelings you had to forfeit to win your dad's approval. (Criterion 2) I can help you with this, but you must consider that your father's message was wrong, because it was. (Criterion 3)

Example Response to Advanced Client Statement 4

I imagine your mom would be pleased. You have achieved a lot, and I'm sure the university is grateful for your contributions. And while this is all very impressive, I sense that the part of you that desperately needs approval takes over. I hope you know that you don't have to prove yourself to me to have my caring and support. (Criterion 1) This is not meant as a criticism. I think you know how much I admire your success. But this is not the part that makes you a lovable person and a person worthy of care. And I wonder if the thought of sharing the normal disappointments and struggles in your relationship causes you to shift into this approval-seeking mode now with me. (Criterion 2) I am happy to acknowledge your accomplishments, but I would like to pay some attention to meeting the needs of that part of you who is hurting and needs to express your struggles too. (Criterion 3)

Example Response to Advanced Client Statement 5

This "I need no one, and I am superior" part of you always tends to show up when I am offering care and concern. (Criterion 1) Makes sense that you would not easily trust someone's caring, given your experiences with a mom who used you as an occasional surrogate for her sense of specialness. Her caring was conditional, and you were made to perform to suit her needs. When you hear the kindness and caring, it is difficult for you to discern that this is "me" and not your mom, to imagine that I could care for you without you having to perform. This is something you've always needed since you were little. (Criterion 2) And while you do pay me for a service, the caring is something I feel, or I don't feel. So that's free and it's genuine. (Criterion 3)

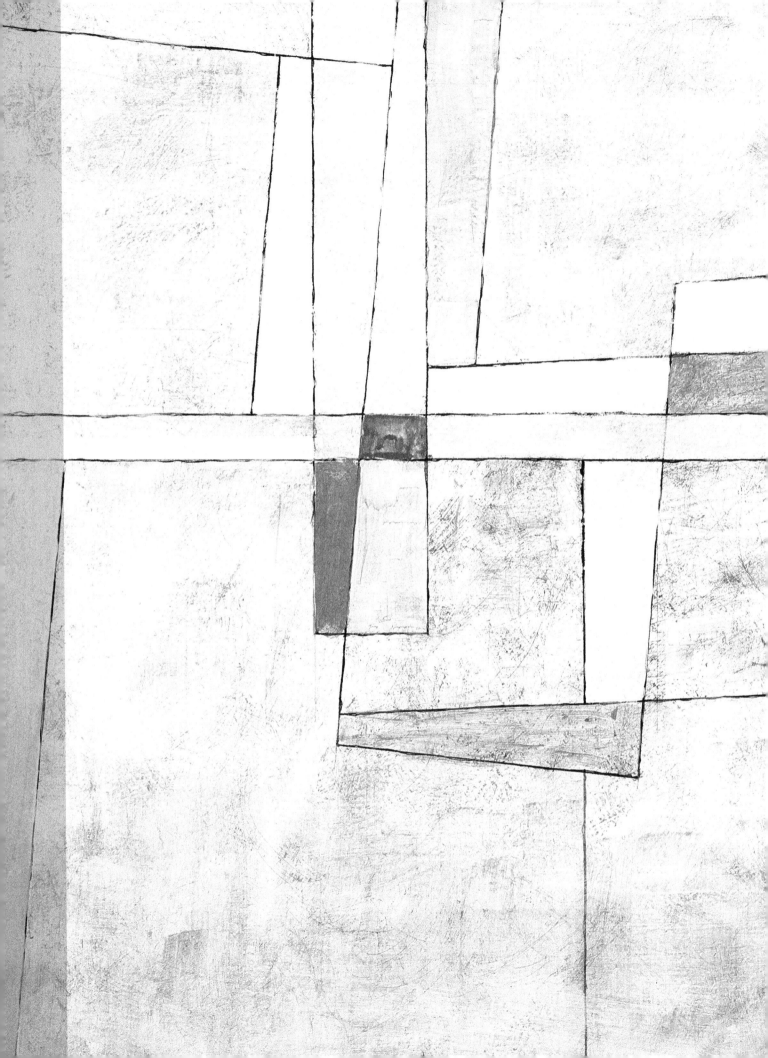

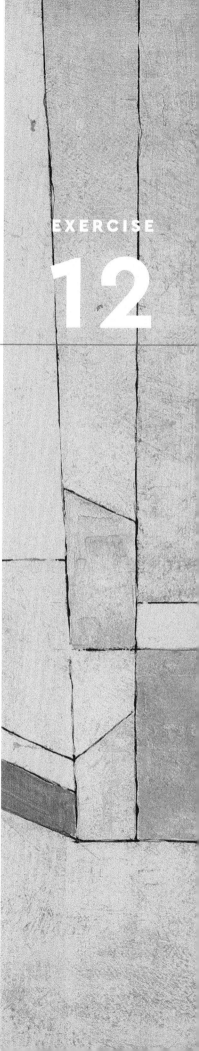

Implementing Behavioral Pattern Breaking Through Homework Assignments

Preparations for Exercise 12

1. Read the instructions in Chapter 2.

2. Download the Deliberate Practice Reaction Form and Deliberate Practice Diary Form at https://www.apa.org/pubs/books/deliberate-practice-schema-therapy (see the "Clinician and Practitioner Resources" tab; also available in Appendixes A and B, respectively).

Skill Description

Skill Difficulty Level: Advanced

Behavioral pattern breaking is an integral component of schema therapy (ST). In this component, the client uses the awareness and self-understanding gained in sessions to affect behavior changes that better meet their needs in healthy adult ways. This is the phase of ST that focuses on strengthening the healthy adult mode. Behavioral pattern breaking is facilitated by the therapist suggesting or assigning appropriate, schema- or mode-based "homework" that the client can try during the week outside of the session to consolidate or advance the therapy work that took place during the session. In ST, many self-help assignments are possible, and they are tailored to fit the unique needs of the client.

In this exercise, we focus on the four most widely used behavioral pattern-breaking assignments in ST. For each client statement, the therapist suggests one of the following assignments for the client to try out during the week, outside the session:

- Assignment 1: Written or audio/video flash cards
- Assignment 2: Writing assignments (e.g., journaling)
- Assignment 3: Schema or mode monitoring
- Assignment 4: Imagery exercises (e.g., safe place imagery)

https://doi.org/10.1037/0000326-014

After this, the therapist provides a brief rationale for why this assignment may be helpful to the client, given the context presented in their statements. The overall message of these interventions is that, through repeated practice, clients can strengthen their healthy adult part and consolidate the work done in session.

SKILL CRITERIA FOR EXERCISE 12

1. Suggest one of the following behavioral pattern-breaking assignments that the client can try during their week:
   - Assignment 1: Written or audio/video flash cards
   - Assignment 2: Writing assignments (e.g., journaling)
   - Assignment 3: Schema or mode monitoring
   - Assignment 4: Imagery exercises (e.g., safe place imagery)

2. Explain how this assignment helps continue the work that took place during the session.

Examples of Implementing Behavioral Pattern Breaking Through Homework Assignments

Example 1

CLIENT: [*Calm*] I'm glad that today we discussed the accuracy of the messages I get from my critic mode. Right now, I feel stronger than the critic, but how can I hang onto this strength?

THERAPIST: We can make an audio flash card that reminds you that the critic is wrong. You can listen to it whenever you hear the critic. (Criterion 1, Assignment 1) In session today, you really felt the limits of the critic's strength when I challenged him playing your healthy adult mode. Repeating that challenge will strengthen your healthy adult mode. (Criterion 2)

Example 2

CLIENT: [*Nervous*] It felt great today to be able to stand up to my dad in the role-play we did. But I don't know whether I'll ever be strong enough to do it in person.

THERAPIST: This week I would like you to write down anything that occurs to you that you would like to say to your dad. You don't need to actually say it to him, just keep a record of it. (Criterion 1, Assignment 2) You stood up to him today, and with practice that ability will get even stronger. It can start with just finding the words to express how you feel or what you need. (Criterion 2)

Example 3

CLIENT: [*Nervous*] I realize because of the work we did today that when my subjugation schema is activated, I surrender and go along with a decision someone important to me makes, even though it is not what I actually want or need. What can I do to make sure that I notice when the schema is activated and make a better choice?

THERAPIST: A way to get started to change that behavior would be to monitor signs that the schema has been triggered so that you remain aware of the pull to subjugate.

(Criterion 1, Assignment 3) That would help to ensure that you stop and consider whether you are meeting your needs like you did in today's session. (Criterion 2)

Example 4

CLIENT: [*Calm*] This was a really helpful session. I know now that I should have had support for expressing my feelings when I was growing up. The imagery rescripting we did let me feel what it would have been like to have that support and how I would think differently about myself and others today.

THERAPIST: That's great! It will be important that you revisit that image a few times this week to reinforce the experience of being supported for expressing how you feel. (Criterion 1, Assignment 4) Doing that will strengthen the experience of support for emotional expression that you felt today in the imagery rescripting we did. (Criterion 2)

INSTRUCTIONS FOR EXERCISE 12

Step 1: Role-Play and Feedback

- The client says the first beginner client statement. The therapist improvises a response based on the skill criteria.
- The trainer (or, if not available, the client) provides brief feedback based on the skill criteria.
- The client then repeats the same statement, and the therapist again improvises a response. The trainer (or client) again provides brief feedback.

Step 2: Repeat

- Repeat Step 1 for all the statements in the current difficulty level (beginner, intermediate, or advanced).

Step 3: Assess and Adjust Difficulty

- The therapist completes the Deliberate Practice Reaction Form (see Appendix A) and decides whether to make the exercise easier or harder or to repeat the same difficulty level.

Step 4: Repeat for Approximately 15 Minutes

- Repeat Steps 1 to 3 for at least 15 minutes.
- The trainees then switch therapist and client roles and start over.

> **Now it's your turn! Follow Steps 1 and 2 from the instructions.**

Remember: The goal of the role-play is for trainees to practice improvising responses to the client statements in a manner that (a) uses the skill criteria and (b) feels authentic for the trainee. **Example therapist responses for each client statement are provided at the end of this exercise. Trainees should attempt to improvise their own responses before reading the example responses.**

BEGINNER-LEVEL CLIENT STATEMENTS FOR EXERCISE 12
Beginner Client Statement 1
[Unsure] It felt great today to be able to stand up to my dad in the role-play we did. However, I don't know whether I will ever be strong enough to do it in person.
Beginner Client Statement 2
[Happy] I really like the things you said to "little me" in the imagery work we did today. I can see how it would help me a lot if I heard those things at times I feel scared.
Beginner Client Statement 3
[Worried] I understand from the Young Schema Questionnaire results we went over today that I have a defectiveness/shame schema from the way I was treated in my childhood, but when it is activated, all I'm aware of is shame.
Beginner Client Statement 4
[Happy] I am glad that today we discussed the accuracy of the messages I get from my critic mode. Right now, I feel stronger than the critic, but how can I hang on to this strength?
Beginner Client Statement 5
[Unsure] I hope I can find the courage to confront my boss just like we practiced today. As you know, I tend to avoid confrontations. We were never allowed to express our disappointments or frustrations in my home. It was too dangerous.

 Assess and adjust the difficulty before moving to the next difficulty level (see Step 3 in the exercise instructions).

INTERMEDIATE-LEVEL CLIENT STATEMENTS FOR EXERCISE 12
Intermediate Client Statement 1
[Hopeful] Here with you today I feel like I might be lovable and not the nuisance that my mom said I was. It is a really good feeling. How do I hang onto it?
Intermediate Client Statement 2
[Curious] I felt relieved today when you told me that I did not have to perform or be perfect to get your attention. However, that was the only way my mother ever noticed me, so I automatically turn into a performer with people today who are important to me. The downside is that I feel like a fake and that no one really knows me. You also said that it is normal to want some attention. How do I remember these things when I am not in therapy?
Intermediate Client Statement 3
[Worried] Today when my abused child mode was activated, I felt afraid of you and it took me a while to hear you saying, "Look at me, I would never hurt you like your mom did." Once I heard you, I could connect with my healthy adult mode. At home when I get triggered with my wife, she says, "Grow up, I am not your mother, you are a 6-foot-tall, physically strong man." What can I do then?
Intermediate Client Statement 4
[Worried] It's really hard to hold onto this important message that you are giving me. It feels so good when you remind me that I have the right to my own choices, opinions, and ideas. But when I am out there in my relationship with my partner, I get triggered so easily, subjugate myself, and sacrifice my needs.
Intermediate Client Statement 5
[Happy] I know I am feeling better about myself because I can finally consider the possibility of leaving this unhealthy relationship. Maybe it's all the mode dialogues we've been doing, having me assert my rights from the healthy advocate part of me and stand up to my rejecting, critical narcissistic parents from my angry child mode and my healthy advocate mode. I feel like I have choices now. I am not staying in this relationship out of fear and desperation.

 Assess and adjust the difficulty before moving to the next difficulty level (see Step 3 in the exercise instructions).

ADVANCED-LEVEL CLIENT STATEMENTS FOR EXERCISE 12

Advanced Client Statement 1

[Happy] Yes, I know I have this terrible defectiveness–shame schema and a harsh demanding critic mode. I quickly escalate into a bully–attack mode and get angry the same way my dad always did. I just want to yell at my wife for not appreciating how hard I am trying and for how sorry I am for the hurt I've caused. I can't seem to catch it early enough to shut it down. But your suggestion that I can use noticing the tension in my neck as an early warning sign is really helpful.

Advanced Client Statement 2

[Determined] I would love to be able to have that relationship with my nephews who love me. But thinking about being nice to them makes me feel like I am giving in to my controlling sister. It's like she wins again. I love the imagery we did where I could imagine spending time with them and being their loving auntie and not paying any attention to my sister's reactions. But I keep anticipating her with her cynical smile as if she is again in charge of my life and I am the pathetic loser. I cannot go back to being abused by her.

Advanced Client Statement 3

[Optimistic] Wow, that was so helpful seeing that link between my anxiety about my daughter's emotional struggles and the terror I felt when I was little and forced to protect my mother from killing herself. I realize that my daughter has grown up without the schemas that I have had to endure. How do I hold onto this?

Advanced Client Statement 4

[Hopeful] The journaling of my interactions with others has really helped. I am beginning to recognize my detached protector mode more easily now. I actually noticed when my partner asked me how I felt about something she said last week, I answered her with a very intellectual response—no feelings. I could see her disappointment and I was able to correct myself. And guess what? It felt good to express my feelings. I wish I could spot the moments where this happens at other times and with other people.

Advanced Client Statement 5

[Curious] It really felt comforting doing the imagery exercise with me in my safe place just before going into that big social event. I felt like I could leave my vulnerable part of me securely tucked away while the adult part of me went into the venue filled with my business associates. Still scary, but I felt like I could do it. My whole life has been an avoidance of my mother-the-critic reminding me that I better not make a fool of myself in front of others. Will that voice ever go away?

 Assess and adjust the difficulty here (see Step 3 in the exercise instructions). If appropriate, follow the instructions to make the exercise even more challenging (see Appendix A).

Example Therapist Responses: Implementing Behavioral Pattern Breaking Through Homework Assignments

Remember: Trainees should attempt to improvise their own responses before reading the example responses. **Do not read the following responses verbatim unless you are having trouble coming up with your own responses!**

EXAMPLE RESPONSES TO BEGINNER-LEVEL CLIENT STATEMENTS FOR EXERCISE 12
Example Response to Beginner Client Statement 1
This week I would like you to write down anything that occurs to you that you would like to say to your dad. You don't need to actually say it to him, just keep a record of it. (Criterion 1, Assignment 2) You stood up to him today, and with practice that ability will get even stronger. It can start with just finding the words to express how you feel or what you need. (Criterion 2)
Example Response to Beginner Client Statement 2
Of course it would, as "little you" like all children needs validation. Fortunately, I recorded my conversation with "little you" today. I will send you the file so you can play it again on your phone whenever you need it. (Criterion 1, Assignment 1) This week you can play it whenever you like so that "little you" can hear those "good parent" messages again. Doing that will reinforce what we did in our session today and take the new messages into your life. (Criterion 2)
Example Response to Beginner Client Statement 3
Those names come from your critic mode being triggered, and it takes you back to your childhood experiences of being called names. We need to find a way for you to fight that critic mode with your healthy adult mode. I suggest that we write out a schema flash card. (Criterion 1, Assignment 1) Whenever you are aware of feeling shame, you can read the flash card over and remember what we discussed today. Doing this will help strengthen your healthy adult mode. (Criterion 2)
Example Response to Beginner Client Statement 4
We can make an audio flash card that reminds you that the critic is wrong. You can listen to it whenever you hear the critic. (Criterion 1, Assignment 1) In session today, you really felt the limits of the critic's strength when I challenged him playing your healthy adult mode. Repeating that challenge will strengthen your healthy adult mode. (Criterion 2)
Example Response to Beginner Client Statement 5
I can make a flash card for you, which reminds you of the words to use. You can read it before you meet with your boss. (Criterion 1, Assignment 1) Having the words in front of you can provide support for your healthy adult mode. (Criterion 2)

EXAMPLE RESPONSES TO INTERMEDIATE-LEVEL CLIENT STATEMENTS FOR EXERCISE 12

Example Response to Intermediate Client Statement 1

You can go back in imagery to how you felt today hearing my validating statements. You can build up an image of being here in my office, what it looks like, the scents and sights and imagine hearing my voice. (Criterion 1, Assignment 4) Revisiting the image of this experience and hearing my words—that I see you as lovable and interesting, just as you are—is a further way to reduce the power of the schema involved. (Criterion 2)

Example Response to Intermediate Client Statement 2

One way would be for us to write flash cards with those messages on it: "You deserve attention and interest just by being yourself," and "It is OK to want and even ask for attention." You could put them on your bathroom mirror so you see them frequently. (Criterion 1, Assignment 1) Doing this will help you remember the relief and peace that you felt in today's session and fight the negative messages. (Criterion 2)

Example Response to Intermediate Client Statement 3

We can make an audio flash card with the messages you need to hear to access your healthy adult mode. You can play that before having serious discussions with your wife. (Criterion 1, Assignment 1) Practicing connecting with your healthy adult mode like you did in today's session will strengthen that part of you and make it easier for you to protect "little you." (Criterion 2)

Example Response to Intermediate Client Statement 4

I am going to make an audio-recorded flash card for you to listen to, repeating what we worked on today. (Criterion 1, Assignment 1) You can listen to my voice, outside of our sessions, guiding you through the process of identifying the trigger and protecting your vulnerable child, making way for you to assert your choices, feelings, and opinions from your healthy adult mode just like I did in today's session. (Criterion 2)

Example Response to Intermediate Client Statement 5

I can see this too, and I am so proud of you! Let's have you continue to monitor these modes this week as you will be facing some tough decisions in the mediation session with your partner. Pay close attention so you can intervene when you see any of the signs of slipping into your self-doubting, subjugated, surrendering mode and step away for a moment to catch your breath and shift into your healthy adult mode. (Criterion 1, Assignment 3) You had no choice as a little child of narcissistic parents. You were sadly held captive by their demands and emotional neglect. You realized in today's session that you can now make your own choices and get your needs met based on you. (Criterion 2)

EXAMPLE RESPONSES TO ADVANCED-LEVEL CLIENT STATEMENTS FOR EXERCISE 12

Example Response to Advanced Client Statement 1

It is important that you continue to slow down and notice where you are experiencing this sensation in your body. This week I would like you to monitor your modes each day. Just scan your body and notice moments when you feel that sensation. (Criterion 1, Assignment 3) This will alert you to take a few minutes to be with your hurting and shamed little boy like it did in today's session. He needs some comfort and empathy during these times to prevent the shift into your "fight" mode. (Criterion 2)

Example Response to Advanced Client Statement 2

I will audio record the imagery exercise for you to listen to during the week. I want you to continue to focus on the strength and empowerment you feel when you are with your nephews as a healthy adult. (Criterion 1, Assignment 4) "Little you" was powerless when it came to your sister, but the imagery we did today reminded you that you are a grown woman who has power and resourcefulness now. You are no longer at the mercy of your sister, and your nephews are also young adults who would love to have a relationship with their favorite auntie. (Criterion 2)

Example Response to Advanced Client Statement 3

For now, I would like you to try to connect with "little you" each day in your journaling, in your images, and in your breathing exercises, reminding her that she is safe now and she is not responsible, and she has the right to be angry for being put in such a terrible position. (Criterion 1, Assignment 2) This will continue the work we did today to unburden that little girl in you who was given such an unfair and unrealistic role as a child. Your daughter is struggling as many teens do, but she has a loving and protective mom who will support her. (Criterion 2)

Example Response to Advanced Client Statement 4

Bravo! Good for you. Let's see if we can identify, from your journaling, the words, phrases, and experiences that lead to this awareness of your detached mode. And let's have you zoom in on this awareness in your continued journaling. (Criterion 1, Assignment 2) There are clearly schema-triggering moments that can lead to feelings of discomfort and detachment. You began to uncover these links today, and journaling is a way to continue that work. (Criterion 2)

Example Response to Advanced Client Statement 5

Yes, you did beautiful work securing your vulnerable child. How about you make a daily practice of this exercise? (Criterion 1, Assignment 4) Over time, doing this will weaken that voice of your internalized mother-critic as your healthy adult secures the vulnerable child like you did today and engages in more social situations. Eventually you might even be able to bring your playful child into some of these interactions. This is a lovely part of you. (Criterion 2)

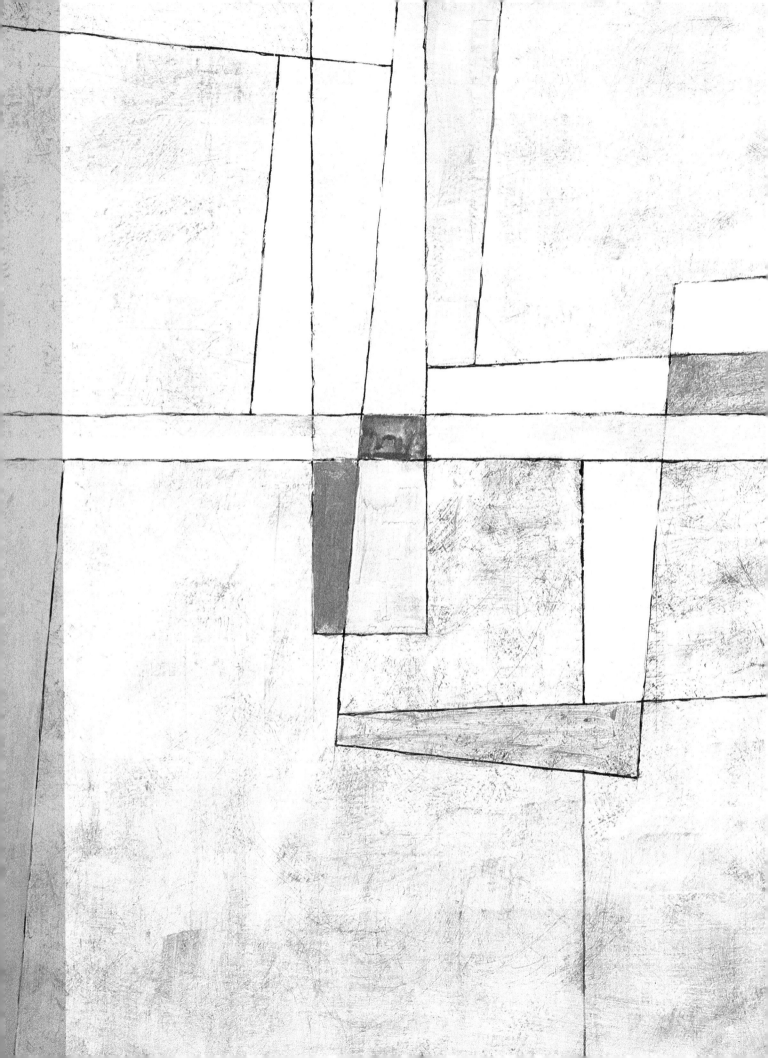

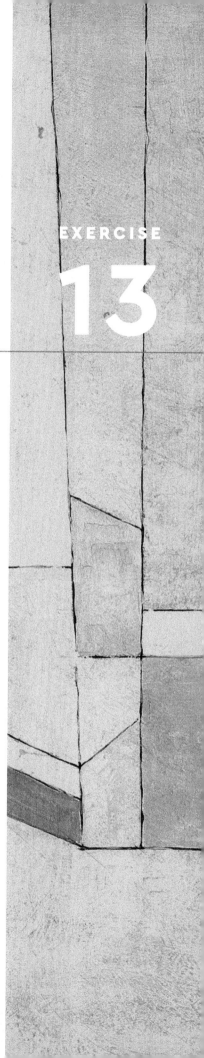

Annotated Schema Therapy Practice Session Transcript

It is now time to put all the skills you have learned together! This exercise presents a transcript from one of Wendy Behary's typical therapy sessions. Therapist statements are annotated to indicate which schema therapy skill from Exercises 1 through 12 is used. This transcript provides an example of how therapists can interweave many schema therapy skills in response to clients.

Instructions

As in the previous exercises, one trainee can play the client while the other plays the therapist. As much as possible, the trainee who plays the client should try to adopt an authentic emotional tone as if they were a real client. The first time through, both partners can read verbatim from the transcript. After one complete run-through, try it again. This time, the client can read from the script, while the therapist can improvise to the degree that they feel comfortable. At this point, you may also want to reflect on it with a supervisor and go through it again. Before you start, it is recommended that both therapist and client read the entire transcript through on your own, until the end. The purpose of the sample transcript is to give trainees the opportunity to try out what it is like to offer schema therapy responses in a sequence that mimics live therapy sessions.

Annotated Schema Therapy Transcript

THERAPIST 1: Nice to see you today. How have you been doing since we last saw each other?

CLIENT 1: Hi. Well . . . I'm still struggling with sleep and arguing with my coworkers even when they are being kind to me. It's been happening ever since I got my divorce. I've come to realize that no matter how much I try, I can't seem to let anyone care for me. I guess that's my pattern.

https://doi.org/10.1037/0000326-015

THERAPIST 2: This feels right to me. This is one of the main things we've been working on. It's great that you're more aware of this pattern, so we can continue to work on it. (Skill 1: Understanding and Attunement)

CLIENT 2: Yeah, that'd be good . . .

THERAPIST 3: And you were also telling me last time that you had a pretty tough upbringing that helped explain this pattern . . .

CLIENT 3: Oh yeah. . . . It's like I came into the world expected to be an adult. I had to learn to bury my needs to care for myself and my little brother. From the time I was little, I was told I had to be tough and competitive.

THERAPIST 4: Right, you grew up with these messages to bury or ignore your needs.

CLIENT 4: [*anxious*] Honestly, even talking about it here seems weird. I never really focused on "my" things, if you get what I mean. Maybe that sounds stupid?

THERAPIST 5: Not at all! I can imagine that perhaps as you anticipate sharing your pain, it's upsetting and maybe even a little scary? All feelings are welcome here. (Skill 1: Understanding and Attunement)

CLIENT 5: [*relaxes*] Okay, thanks. But yeah, if I was going to have any value in this world, any needs were seen as a sign of weakness. And I was also weak if someone else needed to care for me. So yeah, I was better off not having any needs.

THERAPIST 6: Right. . . . And yet, all children have needs, even if they are told to ignore them. You know, this pattern you're describing is what we call a schema. It developed in part because of your childhood experiences and early unmet needs. This schema leads to strong beliefs and expectations that have followed you into your current adult life, like this belief that if you allow someone to care for you, it will mean you are weak. (Skill 3: Schema Education: Beginning to Understand Current Problems in Schema Therapy Terms)

CLIENT 6: A schema? I remember we talked about it last week . . .

THERAPIST 7: Yes. Think of it as a pervasive theme or pattern in your life, usually developed in childhood or adolescence. For example, in our sessions, you've been describing this recurring pattern of ignoring your own needs and not letting others care for you. How do you think your upbringing contributed to this pattern? For instance, did your parents play a role here? (Skill 3: Schema Education)

CLIENT 7: Well, my parents had very high expectations for me. My mother focused all her attention on my academic achievements and my father on my athletic abilities. So my dad would make fun of me . . . and my mother would ignore me. If I showed fear or if I made a mistake, they compared me to my older brother, who they both called "the superhero."

THERAPIST 8: Wow. . . . You know, all children need to know that their feelings matter. To be accepted and loved when they are happy, scared, angry, sad, or when they make a mistake. You were made to feel as if you were bad when you felt scared or worried. (Skill 4: Linking Unmet Needs, Schema, and Presenting Problem) Is that right?

CLIENT 8: Yeah. Anything other than shutting up and winning at stuff was seen as a negative. Frankly, I've sometimes wondered why they even bothered having a second kid. I remember as a kid being really careful about what I said, how I said it, and when I said it.

THERAPIST 9: Kind of like walking on eggshells, emotionally?

CLIENT 9: Oh, definitely. It was like I was always seconds away from again proving what a little shit I was to them. So, to your point, of course I couldn't go up to them and express feelings or needs. The very idea that I should depend on my parents was absolutely foreign when I was growing up. It was "do well, or shut up."

THERAPIST 10: Am I hearing you right that you then grew up with a basic sense that you were in some way defective, not good enough?

CLIENT 10: Sure.

THERAPIST 11: So your early upbringing really consolidated this negative sense of self, and led to the development of what we call a defectiveness/shame schema. Given your early experiences, when this schema is activated, you feel that you can't express your feelings or allow someone else to comfort you. Again, this schema is a very strong emotional belief that was developed early on and now still has a powerful hold over you. (Skill 4: Linking Unmet Needs, Schema, and Presenting Problem)

CLIENT 11: Yes, that makes sense. But . . . it's in the past and I must get over it and stop whining about things that can't be changed. I've already sabotaged my marriage. I really must get over it now. I keep acting like a loser and making a big deal out of everything. Feeling sorry for myself is pathetic. I should just be able to get on with my life.

THERAPIST 12: Wow, that's a harsh self-criticism, just as you started to share some important feelings and insights. Sounds like you've just shifted into a mode as your schema was being triggered. I think we probably don't have to wonder where this inner critical voice may be coming from. (Skill 5: Education About Maladaptive Schema Modes)

CLIENT 12: I just need to learn to be tougher and focus on what matters, my work, and my success. My father was probably right. I need to stop jeopardizing my career and life with all this stupid worry. I can be such a loser, loser, loser . . .

THERAPIST 13: I hear your inner critic loud and clear! Your critic's statements are very harsh and unfair to you. It sounds like you are hearing your dad's voice calling you a "loser." (Skill 7: Identifying the Presence of the Demanding/Punitive Inner Critic Mode)

CLIENT 13: Yeah, I can hear it too. You're right, that's what he often called me. . . . It's just that I actually really love my dad, but then I remember all the times he was horrible to me. . . . So it's hard to make sense of it sometimes . . .

THERAPIST 14: Yeah, I hear that it is very confusing to have such strong conflicted feelings. You love your dad, but you were also badly hurt. I want you to know that you have my support in this, and I know it is difficult. Let's look together at the details of what happened and help you process these complex feelings. (Skill 1: Understanding and Attunement)

CLIENT 14: I guess the part I get most confused about is what a "normal" childhood should look like. I know my dad wasn't that great to me, but it's hard to picture anything different after having been treated like shit for so many years. And again, I just end up feeling like a loser . . .

THERAPIST 15: Every child needs to feel cherished and accepted by their caregivers. This internal critic that showed up, your father's voice and early message, is harsh and terribly unfair, and it's also not true. (Skill 10: Limited Reparenting for the Demanding/Punitive Inner Critic Mode)

CLIENT 15: I know a part of me believes that . . . that he was unfair . . .

THERAPIST 16: Oh?

CLIENT 16: I remember one time telling him off. It probably only happened that one time, when I was around 15. He was going on about what a disappointment I was, how I was needy and didn't deserve all the benefits I had in life. Something in me just flipped. I told him I didn't get what he got out of humiliating me and that I just wanted him to leave me alone if he only had nasty things to say. I remember shaking uncontrollably while doing it . . .

THERAPIST 17: Wow! Good for you! Your healthy adult mode was able to advocate for your rights. I know that must have been so hard with someone like your dad. I really admire that part of you that you just described, even if your parents didn't support it. It's your right to be respected just as you are and to fight for your needs. (Skill 2: Supporting and Strengthening the Healthy Adult Mode)

CLIENT 17: [sad] Thanks. . . . Well . . . [suddenly flat, detached] okay, listen, I really do get what you're saying. But I'm upset about losing my marriage, arguing with my coworkers, and feeling like a failure. And I don't know why I have to talk about these upsetting things. I don't see how it helps me to feel better and to be productive. You know, again, I can just imagine my dad if he knew I was talking to you. He would be laughing at me saying that nothing good comes from self-pity and that therapists just want to make you cry because that's what they are trained to do.

THERAPIST 18: There's that tough part of you again. The part that shuts down all connection to reasonable emotions and becomes critical of therapy and my motivations. I noticed that you sounded sad for a moment and then switched, dismissing the feelings you shared. I think a coping mode was triggered. Are you aware of this shift? (Skill 6: Recognizing the Mode Shifts of the Maladaptive Coping Modes)

CLIENT 18: Yeah, I guess. . . . [softens] It's just so hard to see what I can do to overcome this . . .

THERAPIST 19: It's not your fault. As you said, your father had you believe that you are wasting time when you allow yourself to experience difficult emotions and that you should not trust anyone who wants to know you in this deep and personal way. This may also be why you are still struggling with sleep and having trouble with your coworkers. The sadness of the divorce is valid and painful and needs a space to be felt and grieved, just like all the feelings you had to forfeit to win your dad's approval. I can help you with this, but you must consider that your father's message was wrong, because it was. (Skill 11: Limited Reparenting for the Maladaptive Coping Modes: Empathic Confrontation)

CLIENT 19: Thanks. . . . I actually like that you're so direct about that! [laughs] I think you're right, it's all connected.

[From here, the therapist and client spend the majority of the session engaging in imagery work focused on the client's defectiveness/shame schema and inner critic. The following exchanges come after this piece of imagery work is done.]

CLIENT 58: Wow . . . yeah, I'm much more aware that I have this terrible schema and a harsh critic mode. I quickly escalate and get angry the same way my dad always did. I never really realized that connection so clearly until we worked on it today . . .

THERAPIST 59: Right. I'm happy to work on this more with you, to see if we can help heal this schema and help you have better relationships.

CLIENT 59: I guess one of my main problems is that sometimes I can't seem to catch my escalation early enough to shut it down. But your suggestion that I can use noticing the tension in my neck as an early warning sign is really helpful.

THERAPIST 60: It is important that you continue to slow down and notice where you are experiencing this sensation in your body. This week I would like you to monitor your modes each day. Just scan your body and notice moments when you feel that sensation. This will alert you to take a few minutes to be with your hurting and shamed little boy like it did in today's session. He needs some comfort and empathy during these times to prevent the shift into your "fight" mode. (Skill 12: Implementing Behavioral Pattern Breaking Through Homework Assignments)

CLIENT 60: Thanks, I think you're right. I'll try that.

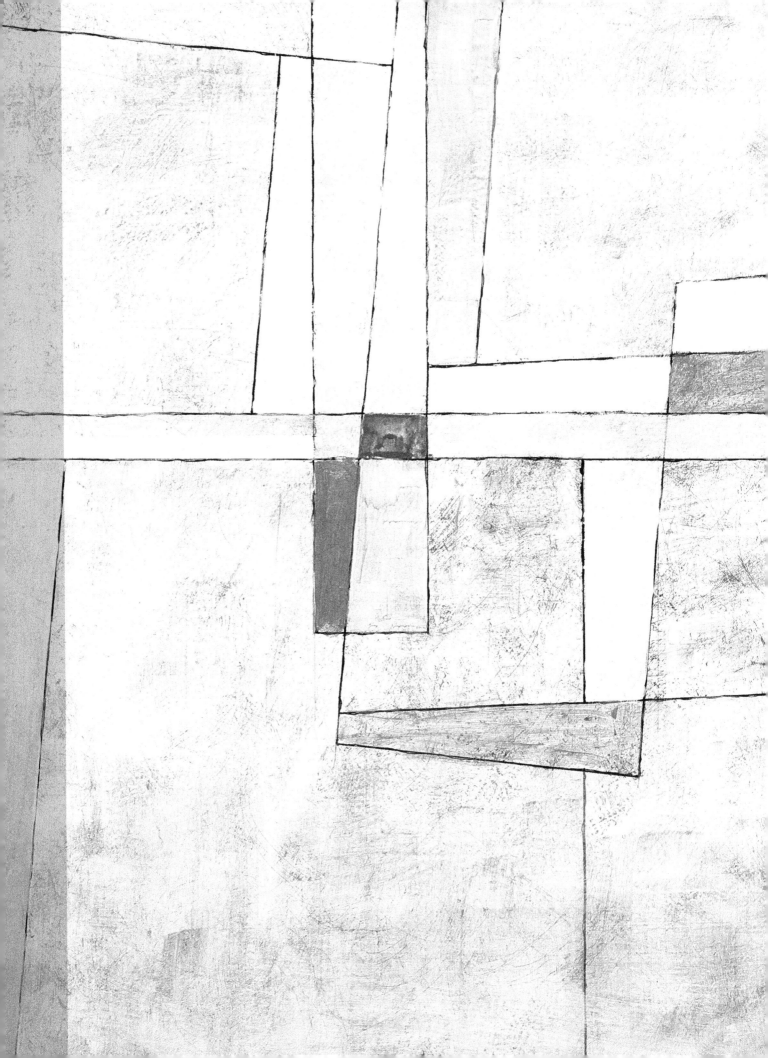

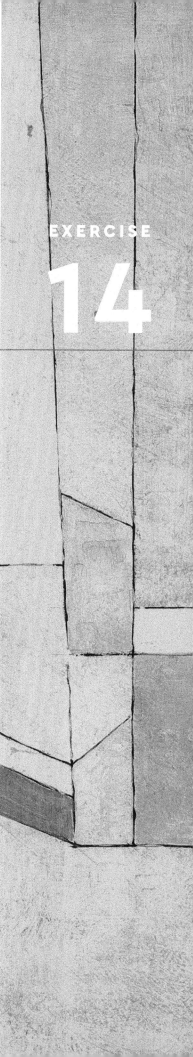

Mock Schema Therapy Sessions

In contrast to highly structured and repetitive deliberate practice exercises, a mock schema therapy (ST) session is an unstructured and improvised role-play therapy session. Like a jazz rehearsal, mock sessions let you practice the art and science of *appropriate responsiveness* (Hatcher, 2015; Stiles & Horvath, 2017), putting your psychotherapy skills together in a way that is helpful to your mock client. This exercise outlines the procedure for conducting a mock ST session. It offers different client profiles you may choose to adopt when enacting a client.

Mock sessions are an opportunity for trainees to practice the following:

- using psychotherapy skills responsively
- navigating challenging choice-points in therapy
- choosing which interventions to use
- tracking the arc of a therapy session and the overall big-picture therapy treatment
- guiding treatment in the context of the client's preferences
- determining realistic goals for therapy in the context of the client's capacities
- knowing how to proceed when the therapist is unsure, lost, or confused
- recognizing and recovering from therapeutic errors
- discovering your personal therapeutic style
- building endurance for working with real clients

Mock ST Session Overview

For the mock session, **you will perform a role-play of an initial therapy session**. As is true with the exercises to build individual skills, the role-play involves three people: One trainee role-plays the therapist, another trainee role-plays the client, and a trainer (a professor or a supervisor) observes and provides feedback. This is an open-ended role-play, as is commonly done in training. However, this differs in two important ways

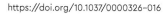

https://doi.org/10.1037/0000326-016

Deliberate Practice in Schema Therapy, by W. T. Behary, J. M. Farrell, A. Vaz, and T. Rousmaniere

from the role-plays used in more traditional training. First, the therapist will use their hand to indicate how difficult the role-play feels. Second, the client will attempt to make the role-play easier or harder to ensure the therapist is practicing at the right difficulty level.

Preparation

1. Download the Deliberate Practice Reaction Form and the Deliberate Practice Diary Form from the "Clinician and Practitioner Resources" tab at https://www.apa.org/pubs/books/deliberate-practice-schema-therapy (also available in Appendixes A and B, respectively). Every student will need their own copy of the Deliberate Practice Reaction Form on a separate piece of paper so they can access it quickly.

2. Designate one student to role-play the therapist and one student to role-play the client. The trainer will observe and provide corrective feedback.

Mock ST Session Procedure

1. The trainees will role-play an initial (first) therapy session. The trainee role-playing the client selects a client profile from the end of this exercise.

2. Before beginning the role-play, the therapist raises their hand to their side, at the level of their chair seat (see Figure E14.1). They will use this hand throughout the role-play to indicate how challenging it feels to them to help the client. Their starting hand level

FIGURE E14.1. Ongoing Difficulty Assessment Through Hand Level

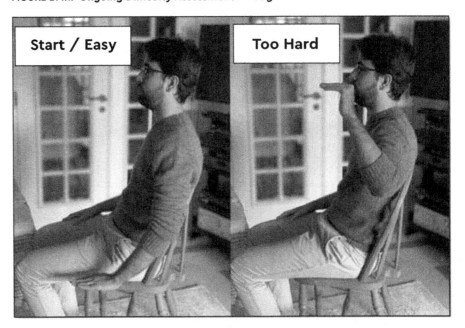

Note. Left: Start of role-play. Right: Role-play is too difficult. From *Deliberate Practice in Emotion-Focused Therapy* (p. 156), by R. N. Goldman, A. Vaz, and T. Rousmaniere, 2021, American Psychological Association (https://doi.org/10.1037/0000227-000). Copyright 2021 by the American Psychological Association.

(chair seat) indicates that the role-play feels easy. By raising their hand, the therapist indicates that the difficulty is rising. If their hand rises above their neck level, it indicates that the role-play is too difficult.

3. The therapist begins the role-play. The therapist and client should engage in the role-play in an improvised manner, as they would engage in a real therapy session. The therapist keeps their hand out at their side throughout this process. (This may feel strange at first!)

4. Whenever the therapist feels that the difficulty of the role-play has changed significantly, they should move their hand up if it feels more difficult and down if it feels easier. If the therapist's hand drops below the seat of their chair, the client should make the role-play more challenging; if the therapist's hand rises above their neck level, the client should make the role-play easier. Instructions for adjusting the difficulty of the role-play are described in the "Varying the Level of Challenge" section.

5. The role-play continues for at least 15 minutes. The trainer may provide corrective feedback during this process if the therapist gets significantly offtrack. However, trainers should exercise restraint and keep feedback as short and tight as possible, as this will reduce the therapist's opportunity for experiential training.

6. After the role-play is finished, the therapist and client switch roles and begin a new mock session.

7. After both trainees have completed the mock session as a therapist, the trainees and the trainer discuss the experience.

Note to Therapists

Remember to be aware of your vocal quality. Match your tone to the client's presentation. Thus, if the clients present vulnerable, soft emotions behind their words, soften your tone to be soothing and calm. If clients, on the other hand, are aggressive and angry, match your tone to be firm and solid. If you choose responses that are prompting client exploration, such as linking unmet needs, schema, and presenting problem, remember to adopt a more querying, exploratory tone of voice.

Varying the Level of Challenge

If the therapist indicates that the mock session is too easy, the person enacting the role of the client can use the following modifications to make it more challenging (see also Appendix A):

- The client can improvise with topics that are more evocative or make the therapist uncomfortable, such as expressing currently held strong feelings (see Figure A.2).
- The client can use a distressed voice (e.g., angry, sad, sarcastic) or unpleasant facial expression. This increases the emotional tone.
- Blend complex mixtures of opposing feelings (for example, love and rage).
- Become confrontational, questioning the purpose of therapy or the therapist's fitness for the role.

If the therapist indicates that the mock session is too hard:

- The client can be guided by Figure A.2 to
    - present topics that are less evocative,
    - present material on any topic but without expressing feelings, or
    - present material concerning the future or the past or events outside therapy.
- The client can ask the questions in a soft voice or with a smile. This softens the emotional stimulus.
- The therapist can take short breaks during the role-play.
- The trainer can expand the feedback phase by discussing ST theory.

Mock Session Client Profiles

Following are six client profiles for trainees to use during mock sessions, presented in order of difficulty. The choice of client profile may be determined by the trainee playing the therapist, the trainee playing the client, or assigned by the trainer.

The most important aspect of role-plays is for trainees to convey the emotional tone indicated by the client profile (e.g., "angry" or "sad"). The demographics of the client (e.g., age, gender) and specific content of the client profiles are not important. Thus, trainees should adjust the client profile to be most comfortable and easy for the trainee to role-play. For example, a trainee may change the client profile from female to male, from 45 to 22 years old, and so on.

Beginner Profile: Processing Grief With a Receptive Client

Laura is a 28-year-old Latinx waitress whose mother died from cancer about 6 months ago. Laura has been experiencing sadness about losing her mother. Her grief is complicated by feelings of anger she has about her mother not being very attentive or loving during Laura's childhood. Laura's mother was very busy when she was growing up, caring for the family while trying to hold multiple jobs; however, Laura still feels her mother was hard on her. She also misses her two siblings, who were forced to go back to Mexico because they were undocumented. Laura wants help processing her grief and anger about her mother.

- **Presenting problems:** Grief, anger, and loneliness
- **Client's goals for therapy:** Laura wants to process her complex feelings about her mother and reconnect with her siblings.
- **Attitude toward therapy:** Laura had good experiences in therapy previously when she was in high school and is optimistic about therapy helping again.
- **Strengths:** Laura is very motivated for therapy and is emotionally open with the therapist.

Beginner Profile: Addressing Loneliness With an Engaged Client

Susan is a 25-year-old African American accountant who recently moved across the country for a new job. While she loves her new job, she has had trouble making friends. She is coming to therapy because she is feeling lonely. She recently went on a date and was disappointed when it didn't go well. She's worried that she will get demoralized and stop trying to make new friends.

- **Presenting problems:** Loneliness, sadness, and demoralization
- **Client's goals for therapy:** Susan wants to build motivation to make more friends and go on more dates.
- **Attitude toward therapy:** Susan has had positive experiences in therapy before. She is hopeful that this therapy will help as well.
- **Strengths:** Susan is emotionally open and motivated to engage in the therapy tasks.

Intermediate Profile: Addressing Anxiety With a Nervous Client

Bob is a 35-year-old White electrician who suffers from extreme anxiety, panic attacks, and shame. He feels like he has been a "loser" his whole life. He was bullied in high school and thinks that people still judge him. He tries to avoid contact with people except through online computer games. He was referred to therapy by his boss, who noticed that Bob would sometimes not show up for work or leave work early. Bob has trouble identifying any of his feelings except anxiety.

- **Presenting problems:** Anxiety, panic attacks, and social isolation

- **Client's goals for therapy:** Bob wants to feel more confident socially so he can engage in work more reliably.

- **Attitude toward therapy:** Bob didn't want to come to therapy because he felt very nervous about it and thinks that the therapist will judge him. Bob's boss convinced him to try therapy.

- **Strengths:** Underneath his anxiety and shame, Bob really wants to connect with other people, including the therapist.

Intermediate Profile: Helping a Sarcastic and Skeptical Client

Jeff is a 45-year-old Asian American engineer who was referred to therapy by his employer because he has been getting angry at work. He is very smart and gets frustrated quickly when his colleagues do not understand his decisions. When he gets frustrated, Jeff is sarcastic or mean. Jeff understands that this is a problem and wants to be more friendly, but he has been unable to change his behavior. He knows that his colleagues do not like him, so he feels socially isolated at work.

- **Presenting problems:** Outbursts of sarcasm and meanness that cover loneliness and social isolation
- **Client's goals for therapy:** Jeff wants to learn how to be more patient and relate better to his colleagues.
- **Attitude toward therapy:** Jeff has never been in therapy before and is skeptical about whether it will help. He came to therapy because his employer asked him to.
- **Strengths:** Jeff honestly wants to be more prosocial.

Advanced Profile: Helping a Very Distrustful Client

Betty is a 27-year-old African American law school graduate student. She wants to become a public defender when she graduates. Betty is the oldest of four siblings. She and her siblings were sexually and physically abused by her father when she was a child. Her father also beat her mother frequently. (Her father is currently in prison for the physical and sexual abuse.) She also feels she has been very hurt and traumatized by systematic racism and discrimination. She has fought hard to achieve her current status. She does not generally trust the system and feels her interests have not been prioritized or protected. Betty feels a lot of anger toward her father, and also toward her mother for not protecting her and her siblings. Betty's youngest sister recently committed suicide due to the abuse. Betty feels very guilty about not protecting her siblings from her father.

- **Presenting problems:** Anger at parents, guilt about not protecting siblings, and grief about her sister's suicide

- **Client's goals for therapy:** Betty wants to resolve her guilt about her sister.

- **Attitude toward therapy:** Betty went to therapy in grade school but had a bad experience: When she told her therapist about her father's abuse, the therapist didn't believe her and told the father what Betty had said. (Betty found out later that the therapist was a friend of the father.) Thus, Betty is very distrustful of therapists, particularly non–African American therapists.

- **Strengths:** Betty is focused and dedicated to improving her mental health. Betty is extremely resilient. She has strong convictions about social justice. She is fiercely loyal to her friends and family.

Advanced Profile: Helping a Client With Mood Lability and Self-Harm

Jane is a 20-year-old European American college student who is having problems in her relationship; she cycles between being deeply in love with her boyfriend and then hating him when he does something that disappoints her, like forgetting her birthday. When Jane is disappointed by her boyfriend, she feels betrayed and abandoned, gets very angry and depressed, and cuts herself. Jane has a similar pattern with her family and friends, where she cycles between liking them a lot and then feeling betrayed and abandoned when they disappoint her.

- **Presenting problems:** Mood lability, self-harm (cutting), and relationship instability

- **Client's goals for therapy:** Jane wants to find stability in herself and her relationships.

- **Attitude toward therapy:** Jane was in therapy before, which was helpful until the therapist disappointed Jane by missing a session, after which Jane felt betrayed and abandoned and quit therapy. Jane is worried that you (her new therapist) may betray or abandon her.

- **Strengths:** Jane is very open to what the therapist says (when she feels safe in therapy).

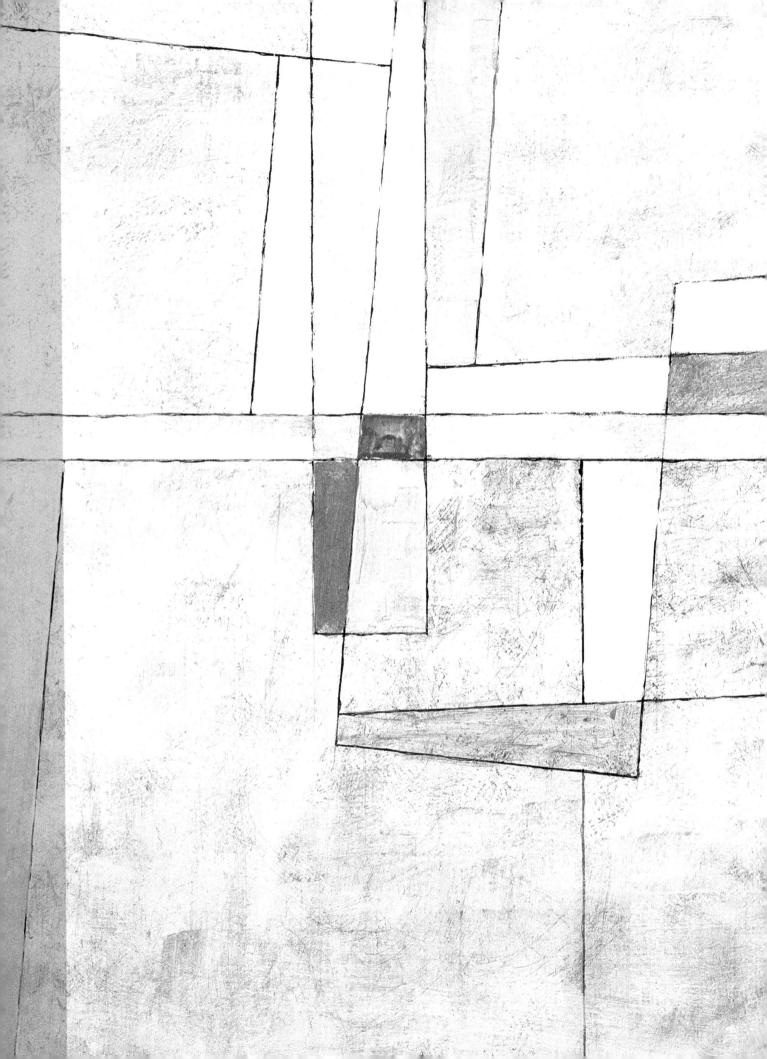

Strategies for Enhancing the Deliberate Practice Exercises

Part III consists of one chapter, Chapter 3, that provides additional advice and instructions for trainers and trainees so that they can reap more benefits from the deliberate practice exercises in Part II. Chapter 3 offers six key points for getting the most out of deliberate practice, guidelines for practicing appropriately responsive treatment, evaluation strategies, methods for ensuring trainee well-being and respecting their privacy, and advice for monitoring the trainer–trainee relationship.

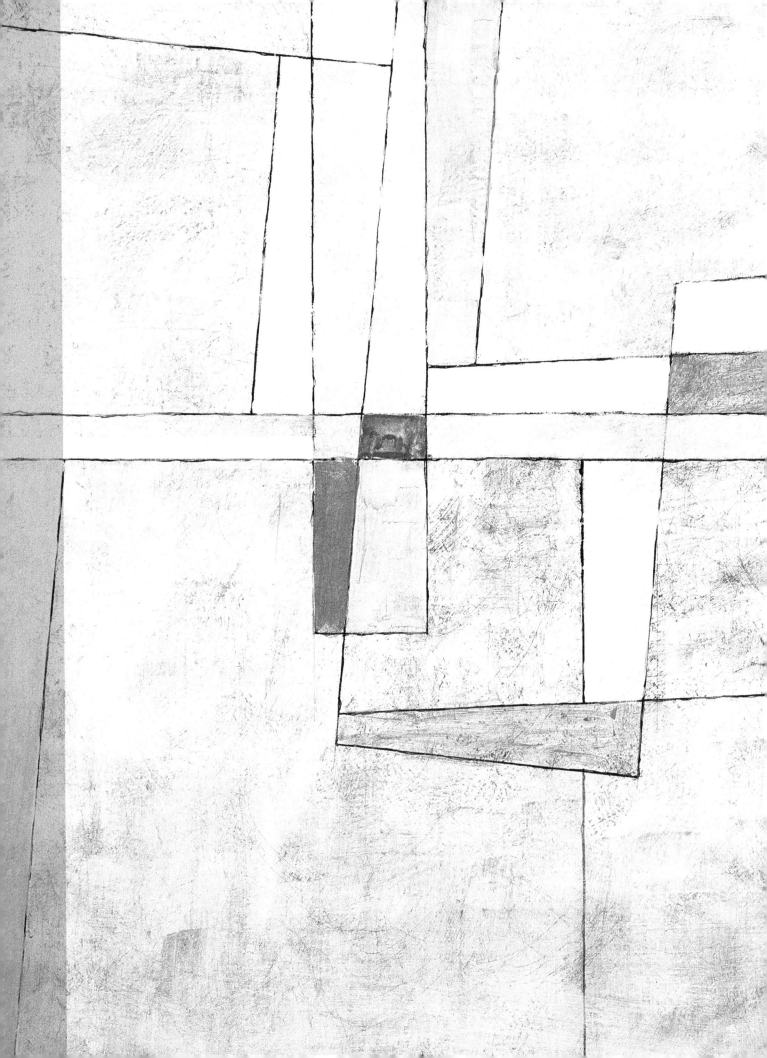

How to Get the Most Out of Deliberate Practice: Additional Guidance for Trainers and Trainees

In Chapter 2 and in the exercises themselves, we provide instructions for completing the deliberate practice exercises. This chapter provides guidance on big-picture topics that trainers will need to successfully integrate deliberate practice into their training program. This guidance is based on relevant research and the experiences and feedback from trainers at more than a dozen psychotherapy training programs who volunteered to test the deliberate practice exercises in this book. We cover topics including evaluation, getting the most from deliberate practice, trainee well-being, respecting trainee privacy, trainer self-evaluation, responsive treatment, and the trainee–trainer alliance.

Six Key Points for Getting the Most From Deliberate Practice

Following are six key points of advice for trainers and trainees to get the most benefit from the schema therapy (ST) deliberate practice exercises. The following advice is gleaned from experiences vetting and practicing the exercises, sometimes in different languages, with many trainees across many countries.

Key Point 1: Create Realistic Emotional Stimuli

A key component of deliberate practice is using stimuli that provoke similar reactions to challenging real-life work settings. For example, pilots train with flight simulators that present mechanical failures and dangerous weather conditions; surgeons practice with surgical simulators that present medical complications with only seconds to respond. Training with challenging stimuli will increase trainees' capacity to perform therapy effectively under stress—for example, with clients they find challenging. The stimuli used for ST deliberate practice exercises are role-plays of challenging client statements in therapy. **It is important that the trainee who is role-playing the client perform the script with appropriate emotional expression and maintain eye contact**

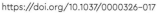

https://doi.org/10.1037/0000326-017

Deliberate Practice in Schema Therapy, by W. T. Behary, J. M. Farrell, A. Vaz, and T. Rousmaniere

with the therapist. For example, if the client statement calls for sad emotion, the trainee should try to express sadness eye-to-eye with the therapist. We offer these suggestions regarding emotional expressiveness:

1. The emotional tone of the role-play matters more than the exact words of each script. Trainees role-playing the client should feel free to improvise and change the words if it will help them be more emotionally expressive. Trainees do not need to stick 100% exactly to the script. In fact, to read from the script during the exercise can sound flat and prohibit eye contact. Rather, trainees in the client role should first read the client statement silently to themselves then, when ready, say it in an emotional manner while looking directly at the trainee playing the therapist. This will help the experience feel more real and engaging for the therapist.

2. Trainees whose first language isn't English may particularly benefit from reviewing and changing the words in the client statement script before each role-play so that they can find words that feel congruent and facilitate emotional expression.

3. Trainees role-playing the client should try to use tonal and nonverbal expressions of feelings. For example, if a script calls for anger, the trainee can speak with an angry voice and make fists with their hands; if a script calls for shame or guilt, the trainee could hunch over and wince; and if a script calls for sadness, the trainee could speak in a soft, deflated voice.

4. If trainees are having persistent difficulties acting believably when following a particular script in the role of client, it may help to first do a "demo round" by reading directly from paper, and then, immediately after, dropping the paper to make eye contact and repeating the same client statement from memory. Some trainees have reported that this helped them "become available as a real clients" and made the role-play feel less artificial. Some trainees did three or four "demo rounds" to get fully into their role as a client.

Key Point 2: Customize the Exercises to Fit Your Unique Training Circumstances

Deliberate practice is less about adhering to specific *rules* than it is about using *training principles*. Every trainer has their own individual teaching style and every trainee their own learning process. Thus, the exercises in this book are designed to be flexibly customized by trainers across different training contexts within different cultures. Trainees and trainers are encouraged to continually adjust exercises to optimize their practice. The most effective training will occur when deliberate practice exercises are customized to fit the learning needs of each trainee and culture of each training site. In our experience with numerous trainers and trainees across many countries, we found that everyone spontaneously customized the exercises for their unique training circumstances. No two trainers followed the exact same procedure. For example:

• One supervisor used the exercises with a trainee who found all the client statements to be too hard, including the "beginner" stimuli. This trainee had multiple reactions in the "too hard" category, including nausea, severe shame, and self-doubt. The trainee disclosed to the supervisor that she had experienced extremely harsh learning environments earlier in her life and found the role-plays to be highly evocative. To help, the supervisor followed the suggestions offered in Appendix A to make the stimuli progressively easier until the trainee reported feeling "good challenge" on the Deliberate Practice Reaction Form. Over many weeks of practice, the trainee developed a sense of safety and was able to practice with more difficult client statements. (Note that if the supervisor had proceeded at the too hard difficulty level, the trainee might have complied while hiding her negative reactions, become emotionally flooded and overwhelmed, leading to withdrawal and thus prohibiting her skill development and risking dropout from training.)

- Supervisors of trainees for whom English was not their first language adjusted the client statements to their own primary language.

- One supervisor used the exercises with a trainee who found all the stimuli to be too easy, including the advanced client statements. This supervisor quickly moved to improvising more challenging client statements from scratch by following the instructions in Appendix A on how to make client statements more challenging.

Key Point 3: Discover Your Own Unique Personal Therapeutic Style

Deliberate practice in psychotherapy can be likened to the process of learning to play jazz music. Every jazz musician prides themselves in their skillful improvisations, and the process of "finding your own voice" is a prerequisite for expertise in jazz musicianship. Yet improvisations are not a collection of random notes but the culmination of extensive deliberate practice over time. Indeed, the ability to improvise is built on many hours of dedicated practice of scales, melodies, harmonies, and so on. Much in the same way, psychotherapy trainees are encouraged to experience the scripted interventions in this book not as ends in themselves but as a means to promote skill in a systematic fashion. Over time, effective therapeutic creativity can be aided, instead of constrained, by dedicated practice in these therapeutic "melodies."

Key Point 4: Engage in a Sufficient Amount of Rehearsal

Deliberate practice uses rehearsal to move skills into procedural memory, which helps trainees maintain access to skills even when working with challenging clients. This only works if trainees engage in many repetitions of the exercises. Think of a challenging sport or musical instrument you learned: How many rehearsals would a professional need to feel confident performing a new skill? Psychotherapy is no easier than those other fields!

Key Point 5: Continually Adjust Difficulty

A crucial element of deliberate practice is training at an optimal difficulty level: neither too easy nor too hard. To achieve this, do difficulty assessments and adjustments with the Deliberate Practice Reaction Form in Appendix A. **Do not skip this step!** If trainees don't feel any of the "good challenge" reactions at the bottom of the Deliberate Practice Reaction Form, then the exercise is probably too easy; if they feel any of the "too hard" reactions, then the exercise could be too difficult for the trainee to benefit. Advanced trainees and therapists may find all the client statements too easy. If so, they should follow the instructions in Appendix A for making client statements harder to make the role-plays sufficiently challenging.

Key Point 6: Putting It All Together With the Practice Transcript and Mock Therapy Sessions

Some trainees may feel a further need for greater contextualization of the individual therapy responses associated with each skill, feeling the need to integrate the disparate pieces of their training in a more coherent manner, with a simulation that mimics a real therapy session. The annotated transcript in Exercise 13 and the mock therapy sessions in Exercise 14 give trainees this opportunity, allowing them to practice delivering different responses sequentially in a more realistic therapeutic encounter.

Responsive Treatment

The exercises in this book are designed to help trainees not only acquire specific skills of ST but also use them in ways that are responsive to each individual client. Across the psychotherapy literature, this stance has been referred to as *appropriate responsiveness*, wherein the therapists exercise flexible judgment, based in their perception of the client's emotional state, needs, and goals, and integrates techniques and other interpersonal skills in pursuit of optimal client outcomes (Hatcher, 2015; Stiles et al., 1998). The effective therapist is responsive to the emerging context. As Stiles and Horvath (2017) argued, a therapist is effective because they are appropriately responsive. Doing the "right thing" may be different each time and means providing each client with an individually tailored response.

Appropriate responsiveness counters a misconception that deliberate practice rehearsal is designed to promote robotic repetition of therapy techniques. Psychotherapy researchers have shown that over-adherence to a particular model while neglecting client preferences reduces therapy effectiveness (e.g., Castonguay et al., 1996; Henry et al., 1993; Owen & Hilsenroth, 2014). Therapist flexibility, on the other hand, has been shown to improve outcomes (e.g., Bugatti & Boswell, 2016; Kendall & Beidas, 2007; Kendall & Frank, 2018). It is important, therefore, that trainees practice their newly learned skills in a manner that is flexible and responsive to the unique needs of a diverse range of clients (Hatcher, 2015; Hill & Knox, 2013). It is thus of paramount importance for trainees to develop the necessary perceptual skills to be able to attune to what the client is experiencing in the moment and form their response based on the client moment-by-moment context.

The supervisor must help the supervisee to attune themselves to the unique and specific needs of the clients during sessions. By enacting responsiveness with the supervisee, the supervisor can demonstrate its value and make it more explicit. In these ways, attention can be given to the larger picture of appropriate responsiveness. Here the trainee and supervisor can work together to help the trainee master not just the techniques but how therapists can use their judgment to put the techniques together to foster positive change. Helping trainees keep this overarching goal in mind while reviewing therapy sessions is a valuable feature of supervision that is difficult to obtain otherwise (Hatcher, 2015).

It is also important that deliberate practice occur within a context of wider ST learning. As noted in Chapter 1, training should be combined with supervision of actual therapy recordings, theoretical learning, observation of competent schema therapists, and personal therapeutic work. When the trainer or trainee determine that the trainee is having difficulty acquiring ST skills, it is important to assess carefully what is missing or needed. Assessment should then lead to the appropriate remedy, as the trainer and trainee collaboratively determine what is needed.

Being Mindful of Trainee Well-Being

Although negative effects that some clients experience in psychotherapy have been well documented (Barlow, 2010), negative effects of training and supervision on trainees has received less attention (Ellis et al., 2014). To support strong self-efficacy, trainers must ensure that trainees are practicing at a correct difficulty level. The exercises in this book feature guidance for frequently assessing and adjusting the difficulty level, so trainees can rehearse at a level that precisely targets their personal skill threshold. Trainers and supervisors must be mindful to provide an appropriate challenge. One risk to trainees that is particularly pertinent to this book occurs when using role-plays that are too difficult. The Deliberate Practice Reaction Form in Appendix A is provided to help trainers ensure that role-plays are done at an appropriate challenge level. Trainers or trainees may be tempted to skip the difficulty assessments and adjustments, out of their motivation to focus on rehearsal to make fast progress and quickly acquire skills. But across all our test sites, we found that skipping the difficulty assessments and adjustments caused more problems and hindered skill acquisition more than any other error. Thus, trainers are advised to remember that **one of their most important responsibilities is to remind trainees to do the difficulty assessments and adjustments.**

Additionally, the Deliberate Practice Reaction Form serves a dual purpose of helping trainees develop the important skills of self-monitoring and self-awareness (Bennett-Levy, 2019). This will help trainees adopt a positive and empowered stance regarding their own self-care and should facilitate career-long professional development.

Respecting Trainee Privacy

The deliberate practice exercises in this book may stir up complex or uncomfortable personal reactions within trainees, including, for example, memories of past traumas. Exploring psychological and emotional reactions may make some trainees feel vulnerable. Therapists of every career stage, from trainees to seasoned therapists with decades of experience, commonly experience shame, embarrassment, and self-doubt in this process. Although these experiences can be valuable for building trainees' self-awareness, it is important that training remain focused on professional skill development and not blur into personal therapy (e.g., Ellis et al., 2014). Therefore, one trainer role is to remind trainees to maintain appropriate boundaries.

Trainees must have the final say about what to disclose or not disclose to their trainer. Trainees should keep in mind that the goal is for the trainee to expand their own self-awareness and psychological capacity to stay active and helpful while experiencing uncomfortable reactions. The trainer does not need to know the specific details about the trainee's inner world for this to happen.

Trainees should be instructed to share only personal information that they feel comfortable sharing. The Deliberate Practice Reaction Form and difficulty assessment process is designed to help trainees build their self-awareness while retaining control over their privacy. Trainees can be reminded that the goal is for them to learn about their own inner world. They do not necessarily have to share that information with trainers or peers (Bennett-Levy & Finlay-Jones, 2018). Likewise, trainees should be instructed to respect the confidentiality of their peers.

Trainer Self-Evaluation

The exercises in this book were tested at a wide range of training sites around the world, including graduate courses, practicum sites, and private practice offices. Although trainers reported that the exercises were highly effective for training, some also said that they felt disoriented by how different deliberate practice feels compared with their traditional methods of clinical education. Many felt comfortable evaluating their trainees' performance but were less sure about their own performance as trainers.

The most common concern we heard from trainers was "My trainees are doing great, but I'm not sure if I am doing this correctly!" To address this concern, we recommend trainers perform periodic self-evaluations along the following five criteria:

1. Observe trainees' work performance.
2. Provide continual corrective feedback.
3. Ensure rehearsal of specific skills is just beyond the trainees' current ability.
4. Ensure that the trainee is practicing at the right difficulty level (neither too easy nor too challenging).
5. Continuously assess trainee performance with real clients.

Criterion 1: Observe Trainees' Work Performance

Determining how well we are doing as trainers means first having valid information about how well trainees are responding to training. This requires that we directly observe trainees practicing skills to provide corrective feedback and evaluation. One risk of deliberate practice is that trainees gain competence in performing therapy skills in role-plays but those skills do not transfer to trainees' work with real clients. Thus, trainers will ideally also have the opportunity to observe samples of trainees' work with real clients, either live or via recorded video. Supervisors and consultants rely heavily—and, too often, exclusively—on supervisees' and consultees' narrative accounts of their work with clients (Goodyear & Nelson, 1997). Haggerty and Hilsenroth (2011) described this challenge:

> Suppose a loved one has to undergo surgery and you need to choose between two surgeons, one of whom has never been directly observed by an experienced surgeon while performing any surgery. He or she would perform the surgery and return to his or her attending physician and try to recall, sometimes incompletely or inaccurately, the intricate steps of the surgery they just performed. It is hard to imagine that anyone, given a choice, would prefer this over a professional who has been routinely observed in the practice of their craft. (p. 193)

Criterion 2: Provide Continual Corrective Feedback

Trainees need corrective feedback to learn what they are doing well, what they are doing poorly, and how to improve their skills. Feedback should be as specific and incremental as possible. Examples of specific feedback are "Your voice sounds rushed. Try slowing down by pausing for a few seconds between your statements to the client" and "That's excellent how you are making eye contact with the client." Examples of vague and nonspecific feedback are "Try to build better rapport with the client" and "Try to be more open to the client's feelings."

Criterion 3: Specific Skill Rehearsal Just Beyond the Trainees' Current Ability (Zone of Proximal Development)

Deliberate practice emphasizes skill acquisition via behavioral rehearsal. Trainers should endeavor not to get caught up in client conceptualization at the expense of focusing on skills. For many trainers, this requires significant discipline and self-restraint. It is simply more enjoyable to talk about psychotherapy theory (e.g., case conceptualization, treatment planning, nuances of psychotherapy models, similar cases the supervisor has had) than watch trainees rehearse skills. Trainees have many questions and supervisors have an abundance of experience; the allotted supervision time can easily be filled sharing knowledge. The supervisor gets to sound smart, while the trainee doesn't have to struggle with acquiring skills at their learning edge. While answering questions is important, trainees' intellectual knowledge about psychotherapy can quickly surpass their procedural ability to perform psychotherapy, particularly with clients they find challenging. Here's a simple rule of thumb: The trainer provides the knowledge, but the behavioral rehearsal provides the skill (Rousmaniere, 2019).

Criterion 4: Practice at the Right Difficulty Level (Neither Too Easy nor Too Challenging)

Deliberate practice involves *optimal strain*: practicing skills just beyond the trainee's current skill threshold so they can learn incrementally without becoming overwhelmed (Ericsson, 2006).

Trainers should use difficulty assessments and adjustments throughout deliberate practice to ensure that trainees are practicing at the right difficulty level. Note that some trainees are surprised by their unpleasant reactions to exercises (e.g., disassociation, nausea, blanking out), and may be tempted to "push through" exercises that are too hard. This can happen out of fear of failing a course, fear of being judged as incompetent, or negative self-impressions by the trainee (e.g., "This shouldn't be so hard"). Trainers should normalize the fact that there will be wide variation in perceived difficulty of the exercises and encourage trainees to respect their own personal training process.

Criterion 5: Continuously Assess Trainee Performance With Real Clients

The goal of deliberately practicing psychotherapy skills is to improve trainees' effectiveness at helping real clients. One of the risks in deliberate practice training is that the benefits will not generalize: Trainees' acquired competence in specific skills may not translate into work with real clients. Thus, it is important that trainers assess the impact of deliberate practice on trainees' work with real clients. Ideally, this is done through triangulation of multiple data points:

1. client data (verbal self-report and routine outcome monitoring data)
2. supervisor's report
3. trainee's self-report

If the trainee's effectiveness with real clients is not improving after deliberate practice, the trainer should do a careful assessment of the difficulty. If the supervisor or trainer feels it is a skill acquisition issues, they may want to consider adjusting the deliberate practice routine to better suit the trainee's learning needs and/or style.

Therapists have traditionally been evaluated from a lens of *process accountability* (Markman & Tetlock, 2000; see also Goodyear, 2015), which focuses on demonstrating specific behaviors (e.g., fidelity to a treatment model) without regard to the impact on clients. We propose that clinical effectiveness is better assessed through a lens tightly focused on client outcomes and that learning objectives shift from performing behaviors that experts have decided are effective (i.e., the competence model) to highly individualized behavioral goals tailored to each trainee's zone of proximal development and performance feedback. This model of assessment has been termed *outcome accountability* (Goodyear, 2015), which focuses on client changes rather than therapist competence, independent of how the therapist might be performing expected tasks.

Guidance for Trainees

The central theme of this book has been that skill rehearsal is not automatically helpful. Deliberate practice must be done well for trainees to benefit (Ericsson & Pool, 2016). In this chapter and in the exercises, we offer guidance for effective deliberate practice. We would also like to provide additional advice specifically for trainees. That advice is drawn from what we have learned at our volunteer deliberate practice test sites around the world. We cover how to discover your own training process, active effort, playfulness and taking breaks during deliberate practice, your right to control your self-disclosure to trainers, monitoring training results, monitoring complex reactions towards the trainer, and your own personal therapy.

Individualized Schema Therapy Training: Finding Your Zone of Proximal Development

Deliberate practice works best when training targets each trainee's personal skill thresholds. Also called the *zone of proximal development*, a term first coined by Vygotsky in reference to developmental learning theory (Zaretskii, 2009), this is the area just beyond the trainee's current ability but that is possible to reach with the assistance of a teacher or coach (Wass & Golding, 2014). **If a deliberate practice exercise is either too easy or too hard, the trainee will not benefit.** To maximize training productivity, elite performers follow a "challenging but not overwhelming" principle: Tasks that are too far beyond their capacity will prove ineffective and even harmful; it is equally true that mindlessly repeating what they can already do confidently will prove fruitless. Because of this, deliberate practice requires ongoing assessment of the trainee's current skill and concurrent difficulty adjustment to consistently target a "good enough" challenge. Thus, if you are practicing Exercise 11 ("Limited Reparenting for the Maladaptive Coping Modes: Empathic Confrontation") and it just feels too difficult, consider moving back to a more comfortable skill, such as Exercise 6 ("Recognizing the Mode Shifts of the Maladaptive Coping Modes").

Active Effort

It is important for trainees to maintain an active and sustained effort while doing the deliberate practice exercises in this book. Deliberate practice really helps when trainees push themselves up to and past their current ability. This is best achieved when trainees take ownership of their own practice by guiding their training partners to adjust role-plays to be as high on the difficulty scale as possible without hurting themselves. This will look different for every trainee. Although it can feel uncomfortable or even frightening, this is the zone of proximal development where the most gains can be made. Simply reading and repeating the written scripts will provide little or no benefit. Trainees are advised to remember that their effort from training should lead to more confidence and comfort in session with real clients.

Stay the Course: Effort Versus Flow

Deliberate practice only works if trainees push themselves hard enough to break out of their old patterns of performance, which then permits growth of new skills (Ericsson & Pool, 2016). Because deliberate practice constantly focuses on the current edge of one's performance capacity, it is inevitably a straining endeavor. Indeed, professionals are unlikely to make lasting performance improvements unless there is sufficient engagement in tasks that are just at the edge of one's current capacity (Ericsson, 2003, 2006). From athletics or fitness training, many of us are familiar with this process of being pushed out of our comfort zones followed by adaptation. The same process applies to our mental and emotional abilities.

Many trainees might feel surprised to discover that deliberate practice for ST feels harder than psychotherapy with a real client. This may be because when working with a real client a therapist can get into a state of *flow* (Csikszentmihalyi, 1997), where work feels effortless. In contrast, effective skill-building tends to be inherently effortful and taxing, often quickly depleting therapists' energy when practicing a particularly challenging task. In such cases, therapists may want to move back to offering response formats with which they are more familiar and feel more proficient and try those for a short time, in part to increase a sense of confidence and mastery.

Discover Your Own Training Process

The effectiveness of deliberate practice is directly related to the effort and ownership trainees exert while doing the exercises. Trainers can provide guidance, but it is important for trainees to learn about their own idiosyncratic training processes over time. This will let them become masters of their own training and prepare for a career-long process of professional development. The following are a few examples of personal training processes trainees discovered while engaging in deliberate practice:

- One trainee noticed that she is good at persisting while an exercise is challenging but also that she requires more rehearsal than other trainees to feel comfortable with a new skill. This trainee focused on developing patience with her own pace of progress.

- One trainee noticed that he can acquire new skills rather quickly, with only a few repetitions. However, he also noticed that his reactions to evocative client statements can jump very quickly and unpredictably from the "good challenge" to "too hard" categories, so he needs to carefully attend to the reactions listed in the Deliberate Practice Reaction Form.

- One trainee described herself as "perfectionistic" and felt a strong urge to "push through" an exercise even when she had anxiety reactions in the "too hard" category, such as nausea and disassociation. This caused the trainee not to benefit from the exercises and potentially become demoralized. This trainee focused on going slower, developing self-compassion regarding her anxiety reactions, and asking her training partners to make role-plays less challenging.

Trainees are encouraged to reflect deeply on their own experiences using the exercises in order to learn the most about themselves and their personal learning processes.

Playfulness and Taking Breaks

Psychotherapy is serious work that often involves painful feelings. However, practicing psychotherapy can be playful and fun (Scott Miller, personal communication, 2017). Trainees should remember that one of the main goals of deliberate practice is to experiment with different approaches and styles of therapy. If deliberate practice ever feels rote, boring, or routine, it probably isn't going to help advance trainees' skill. In this case, trainees should try to liven it up. A good way to do this is to introduce an atmosphere of playfulness. For example, trainees can try the following:

- Use different vocal tones, speech pacing, body gestures, or other languages. This can expand trainees' communication range.

- Practice while simulating being blind (with a cloth) or deaf. This can increase sensitivity in the other senses.

- Practice while standing up or walking around outside. This can help trainees get new perspectives on the process of therapy.

The supervisor can also ask trainees if they would like to take a 5- to 10-minute break between questions, particularly if the trainees are dealing with difficult emotions and are feeling stressed out.

Additional Deliberate Practice Opportunities

This book focuses on deliberate practice methods that involve active, live engagement between trainees and a supervisor. Importantly, deliberate practice can extend beyond these focused training sessions and be used for homework. For example, a trainee might read the client stimuli quietly or aloud and practice their responses independently between sessions with a supervisor. In such cases, it is important for the trainee to say their therapist responses aloud, rather than rehearse silently in one's head. Alternatively, two trainees can practice as a pair, without the supervisor. Although the absence of a supervisor limits one source of feedback, the peer trainee who is playing the client can serve this role, as they can when a supervisor is present. These additional deliberate practice opportunities are intended to take place between focused training sessions with a supervisor. To optimize the quality of the deliberate practice when conducted independently or without a supervisor, we have developed a Deliberate Practice Diary Form that can be found in Appendix B or downloaded from https://www.apa.org/pubs/books/deliberate-practice-schema-therapy (see the "Clinician and Practitioner Resources" tab). This form provides a template for the trainee to record their experience of the deliberate practice activity, and, ideally, it will aid in the consolidation of learning. This form can be used as part of the evaluation process with the supervisor but is not necessarily intended for that purpose, and trainees are certainly welcome to bring their experience with the independent practice into the next meeting with the supervisor.

Monitoring Training Results

While trainers will evaluate trainees using a competency-focused model, trainees are also encouraged to take ownership of their own training process and look for results of deliberate practice themselves. Trainees should experience the results of deliberate practice within a few training sessions. A lack of results can be demoralizing for trainees and can result in trainees applying less effort and focus in deliberate practice. Trainees who are not seeing results should openly discuss this problem with their trainer and experiment with adjusting their deliberate practice process. Results can include client outcomes and improving the trainee's own work as a therapist, their personal development, and their overall training.

Client Outcomes

The most important result of deliberate practice is an improvement in trainees' client outcomes. This can be assessed via routine outcome measurement (Lambert, 2010;

Prescott et al., 2017), qualitative data (McLeod, 2017), and informal discussions with clients. However, trainees should note that an improvement in client outcome due to deliberate practice can sometimes be challenging to achieve quickly, given that the largest amount of variance in client outcome is due to client variables (Bohart & Wade, 2013). For example, a client with severe chronic symptoms may not respond quickly to any treatment, regardless of how effectively a trainee practices. For some clients, an increase in patience and self-compassion regarding their symptoms may be a sign of progress, rather than an immediate decrease in symptoms. Thus, trainees are advised to keep their expectations for client change realistic in the context of their client's symptoms, history, and presentation. It is important that trainees do not try to force their clients to improve in therapy for the trainee to feel like they are making progress in their training (Rousmaniere, 2016).

Trainee's Work as a Therapist

One important result of deliberate practice is change within the trainee regarding their work with clients. For example, trainees at test sites reported feeling more comfortable sitting with evocative clients, more confident addressing uncomfortable topics in therapy, and more responsive to a broader range of clients.

Trainee's Personal Development

Another important result of deliberate practice is personal growth within the trainee. For example, trainees at test sites reported becoming more in touch with their own feelings, increased self-compassion, and enhanced motivation to work with a broader range of clients.

Trainee's Training Process

Another valuable result of deliberate practice is improvement in the trainees' training process. For example, trainees at test sites reported becoming more aware of their personal training style, preferences, strengths, and challenges. Over time, trainees should grow to feel more ownership of their training process. It is also recommended that training to be a psychotherapist is a complex process that occurs over many years. Experienced, expert therapists still report continuing to grow well beyond their graduate school years (Orlinsky & Ronnestad, 2005). Furthermore, training is not a linear process.

The Trainee–Trainer Alliance: Monitoring Complex Reactions Toward the Trainer

Trainees who engage in hard deliberate practice often report experiencing complex feelings towards their trainer. For example, one trainee said, "I know this is helping, but I also don't look forward to it!" Another trainee reported feeling both appreciation and frustration toward her trainer simultaneously. Trainees are advised to remember intensive training they have done in other fields, such as athletics or music. When a coach pushes a trainee to the edge of their ability, it is common for trainees to have complex reactions toward them.

This does not necessarily mean that the trainer is doing anything wrong. In fact, intensive training inevitably stirs up reactions toward the trainer, such as frustration, annoyance, disappointment, or anger that coexist with the appreciations they feel. In fact, if trainees do not experience complex reactions, it is worth considering whether the deliberate practice is sufficiently challenging. But what we asserted earlier about rights to privacy apply here as well. Because professional mental health training is hierarchical and evaluative, trainers should not require or even expect trainees to share complex reactions they may be experiencing toward them. Trainers should stay open to their sharing, but the choice always remains with the trainee.

Trainee's Own Therapy

When engaging in deliberate practice, many trainees discover aspects of their inner world that may benefit from attending their own psychotherapy. For example, one trainee discovered that her clients' anger stirred up her own painful memories of abuse, another trainee found himself disassociating while practicing empathy skills, and another trainee experienced overwhelming shame and self-judgment when she couldn't master skills after just a few repetitions.

Although these discoveries were unnerving at first, they were ultimately beneficial because they motivated the trainees to seek out their own therapy. Many therapists attend their own therapy. In fact, Norcross and Guy (2005) found in their review of 17 studies that about 75% of the more than 8,000 therapist participants have attended their own therapy. Orlinsky and Ronnestad (2005) found that more than 90% of therapists who attended their own therapy reported it as helpful.

QUESTIONS FOR TRAINEES

1. Are you balancing the effort to improve your skills with patience and self-compassion for your learning process?
2. Are you attending to any shame or self-judgment that is arising from training?
3. Are you being mindful of your personal boundaries and also respecting any complex feelings you may have toward your trainers?

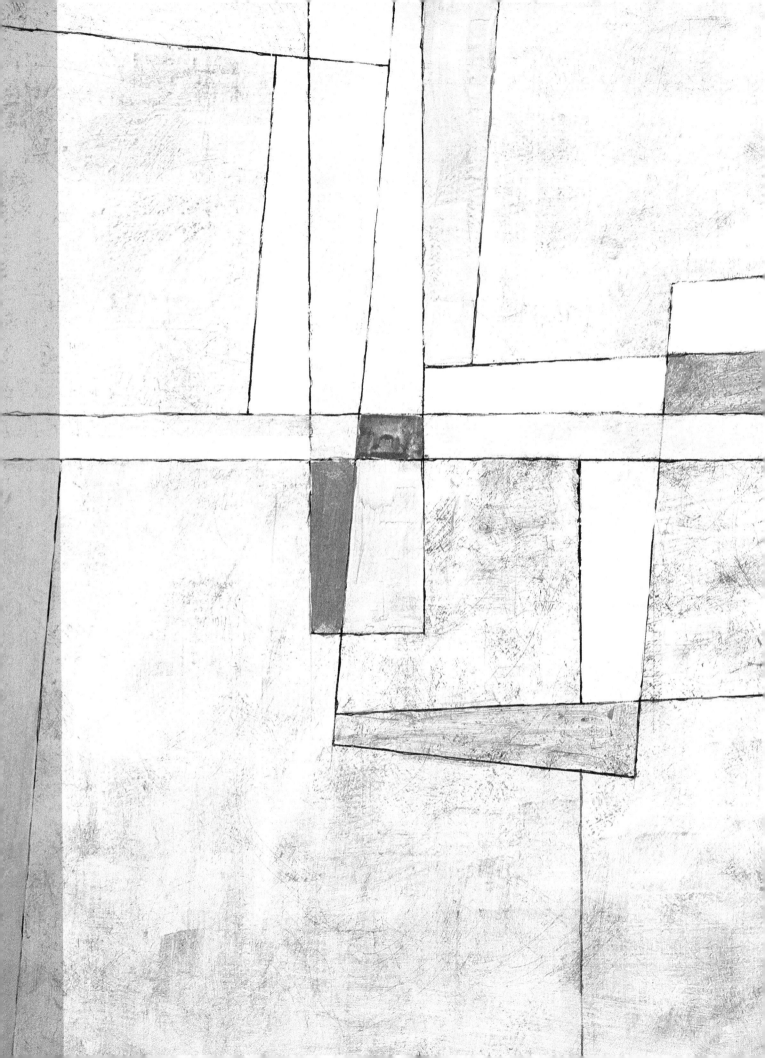

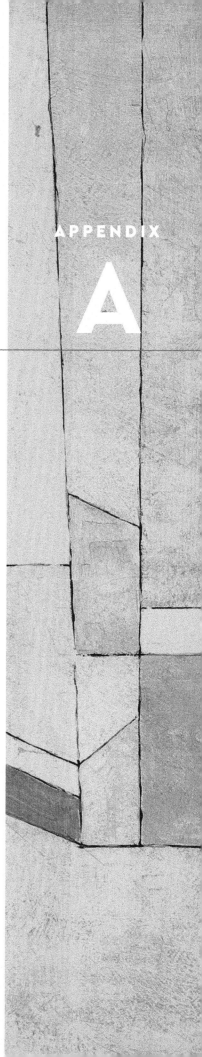

Difficulty Assessments
and Adjustments

Deliberate practice works best if the exercises are performed at a good challenge that is neither too hard nor too easy. To ensure that they are practicing at the correct difficulty, trainees should do a difficulty assessment and adjustment after each level of client statement is completed (beginner, intermediate, and advanced). To do this, use the following instructions and the Deliberate Practice Reaction Form (Figure A.1), which is also available in the "Clinician and Practitioner Resources" tab online (https://www.apa.org/pubs/books/deliberate-practice-schema-therapy). **Do not skip this process!**

How to Assess Difficulty

The therapist completes the Deliberate Practice Reaction Form (Figure A.1). If they

- rate the difficulty of the exercise above an 8 or had any of the reactions in the "Too Hard" column, follow the instructions to make the exercise easier;

- rate the difficulty of the exercise below a 4 or didn't have any of the reactions in the "Good Challenge" column, proceed to the next level of harder client statements or follow the instructions to make exercise harder; or

- rate the difficulty of the exercise between 4 and 8 and have at least one reaction in the "Good Challenge" column, do not proceed to the harder client statements but rather repeat the same level.

Making Client Statements Easier

If the therapist ever rates the difficulty of the exercise above an 8 or has any of the reactions in the "Too Hard" column, use the next level easier client statements (e.g., if you were using advanced client statements, switch to intermediate). But if you already were using beginner client statements, use the following methods to make the client statements even easier:

- The person playing the client can use the same beginner client statements but this time in a softer, calmer voice and with a smile. This softens the emotional tone.

- The client can improvise with topics that are less evocative or make the therapist more comfortable, such as talking about topics without expressing feelings, the future/past (avoiding the here and now), or any topic outside therapy (see Figure A.2).

FIGURE A.1. Deliberate Practice Reaction Form

Question 1: How challenging was it to fulfill the skill criteria for this exercise?

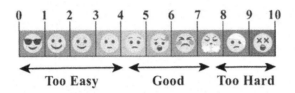

Question 2: Did you have any reactions in "good challenge" or "too hard" categories? (yes/no)					
Good Challenge			**Too Hard**		
Emotions and Thoughts	Body Reactions	Urges	Emotions and Thoughts	Body Reactions	Urges
Manageable shame, self-judgment, irritation, anger, sadness, etc.	Body tension, sighs, shallow breathing, increased heart rate, warmth, dry mouth	Looking away, withdrawing, changing focus	Severe or overwhelming shame, self-judgment, rage, grief, guilt, etc.	Migraines, dizziness, foggy thinking, diarrhea, disassociation, numbness, blanking out, nausea, etc.	Shutting down, giving up

Too Easy	Good Challenge	Too Hard
⬇	⬇	⬇
Proceed to next difficulty level	Repeat the same difficulty level	Go back to previous difficulty level

Note. From *Deliberate Practice in Emotion-Focused Therapy* (p. 180), by R. N. Goldman, A. Vaz, and T. Rousmaniere, 2021, American Psychological Association (https://doi.org/10.1037/0000227–000). Copyright 2021 by the American Psychological Association.

FIGURE A.2. How to Make Client Statements Easier or Harder in Role-Plays

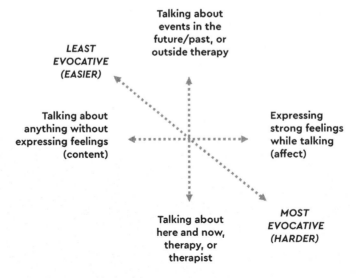

Note. Figure created by Jason Whipple, PhD.

- The therapist can take a short break (5–10 minutes) between questions.

- The trainer can expand the feedback phase by discussing schema therapy or psychotherapy theory and research. This should shift the trainees' focus toward more detached or intellectual topics and reduce the emotional intensity.

Making Client Statements Harder

If the therapist rates the difficulty of the exercise below a 4 or didn't have any of the reactions in the "Good Challenge" column, proceed to next level harder client statements. If you were already using the advanced client statements, the client should make the exercise even harder, using the following guidelines:

- The person playing the client can use the advanced client statements again with a more distressed voice (e.g., very angry, sad, sarcastic) or unpleasant facial expression. This should increase the emotional tone.

- The client can improvise new client statements with topics that are more evocative or make the therapist uncomfortable, such as expressing strong feelings or talking about the here and now, therapy, or the therapist (see Figure A.2).

Note. The purpose of a deliberate practice session is not to get through all the client statements and therapist responses but rather to spend as much time as possible practicing at the correct difficulty level. This may mean that trainees repeat the same statements or responses many times, which is okay, as long as the difficulty remains in the "good challenge" level.

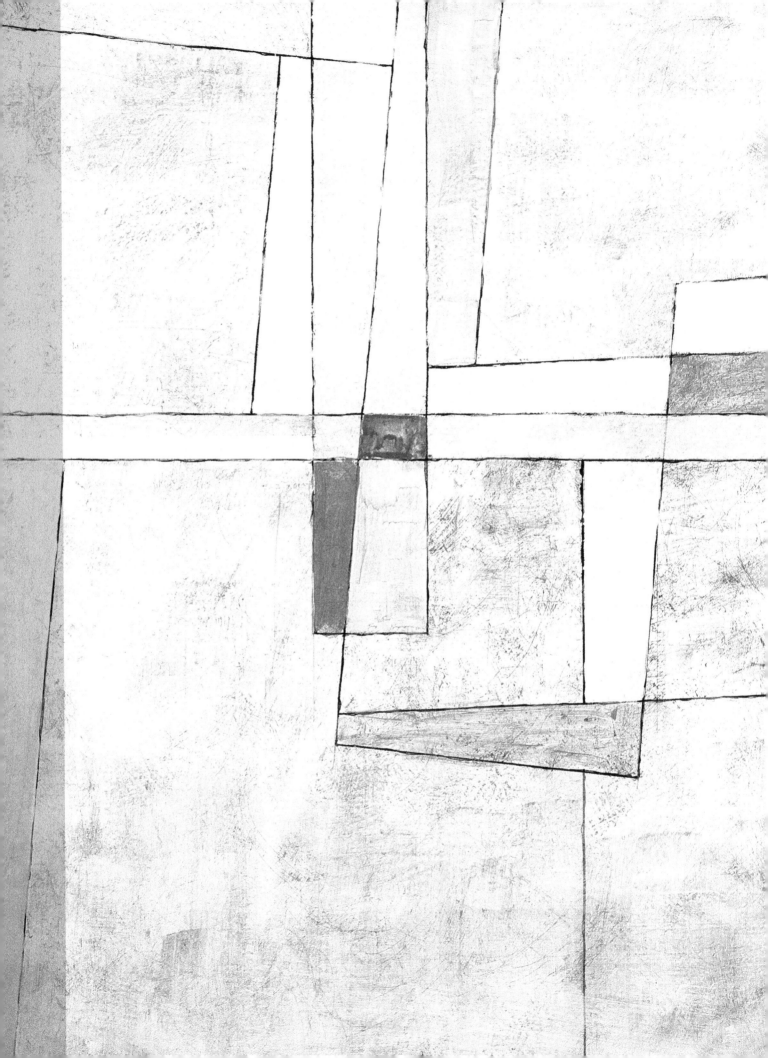

Deliberate Practice Diary Form

To optimize the quality of the deliberate practice, we have developed a Deliberate Practice Diary Form that can also be downloaded from the "Clinician and Practitioner Resources" tab online (https://www.apa.org/pubs/books/deliberate-practice-schema-therapy). This form provides a template for the trainee to record their experience of the deliberate practice activity and, we hope, will aid in the consolidation of learning. This form is not intended to be used as part of the evaluation process with the supervisor.

Deliberate Practice Diary Form

Use this form to consolidate learnings from the deliberate practice exercises. Please protect your personal boundaries by only sharing information that you are comfortable disclosing.

Name: _____ Date: _____

Exercise: _____

Question 1. What was helpful or worked well this deliberate practice session? In what way?

Question 2. What was unhelpful or didn't go well this deliberate practice session? In what way?

Question 3. What did you learn about yourself, your current skills, and skills you'd like to keep improving? Feel free to share any details, but only those you are comfortable disclosing.

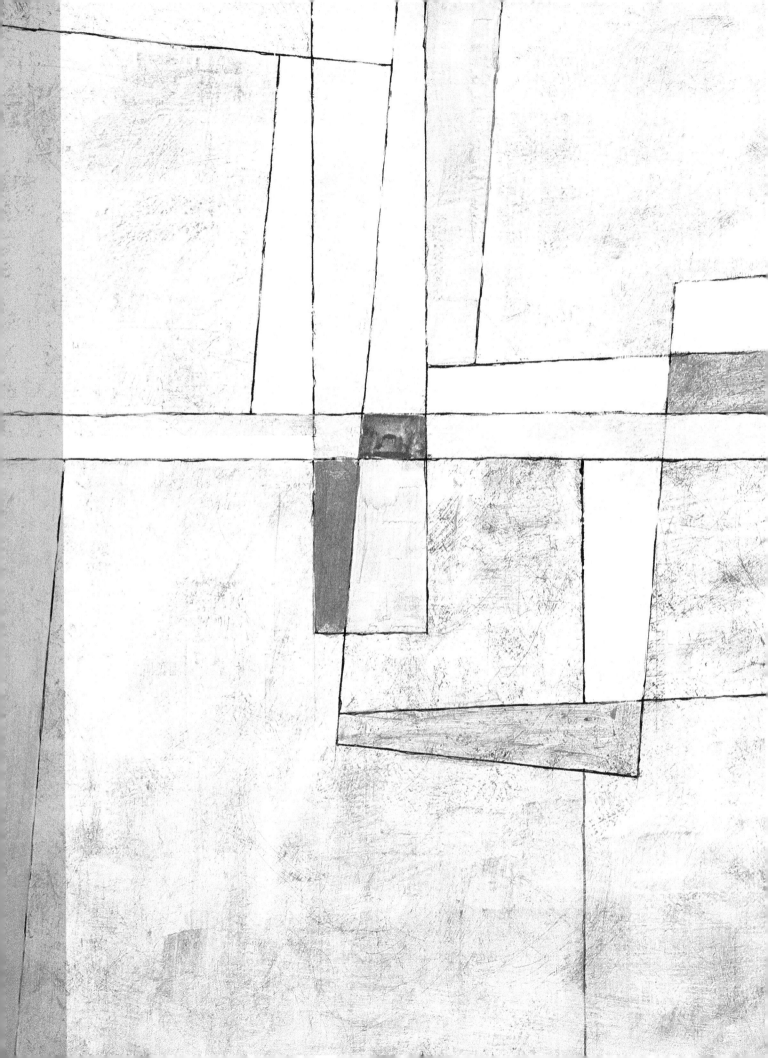

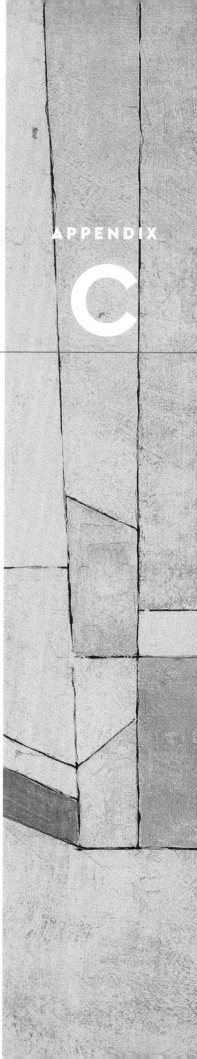

Overview of Schema Therapy Concepts[1]

To get the most out of the exercises in this book, trainees' skill building should be integrated with knowledge of schema therapy (ST) theory. ST is a comprehensive approach in which therapists' interventions are guided by a case conceptualization that rests on several concepts. Therefore, knowledge of these concepts and their relationship to each other is integral to providing effective ST. This appendix provides an overview of some major ST concepts. We recommend that trainees study these and reflect on their importance for clinical practice and, more specifically, their relationship to the skills practiced in this book.

Association of Unmet Core Childhood Needs and Early Maladaptive Schemas

The following is a list of unmet childhood needs, each of which corresponds with a set of early maladaptive schemas.

Unmet Core Childhood Needs

1. Safe attachment: love, validation, protection, acceptance
2. Free expression of emotions and needs
3. Playfulness, spontaneity
4. Autonomy, competence, sense of identity
5. Realistic limits, self-control

Early Maladaptive Schemas

1. Disconnection and rejection

   • Emotional deprivation

   • Defectiveness/shame

   • Mistrust/abuse

   • Social isolation/alienation

   • Abandonment/instability

---

1. Data from Farrell and Shaw (2018).

2. Other directedness
   - Approval seeking/recognition seeking
   - Subjugation
   - Self-sacrifice

3. Overvigilance and inhibition
   - Negativity/pessimism
   - Emotional inhibition
   - Unrelenting standards
   - Punitiveness

4. Impaired autonomy and performance
   - Enmeshment/undeveloped self
   - Failure
   - Vulnerability to harm/illness
   - Dependence/incompetence

5. Impaired limits
   - Insufficient self-control/self-discipline
   - Entitlement/grandiosity

Descriptions of Schema Modes

- **Healthy modes:** Adaptive functioning modes that are associated with a sense of fulfillment and well-being
  - Happy or contented child
  - Healthy adult

- **Demanding/punitive inner critic modes:** Internalized negative aspects from early caregivers. Includes punishing and harsh messages (punitive critic) and setting unreachable expectations and standards (demanding critic)
  - Punitive critic
  - Demanding critic

- **Maladaptive coping modes:** Overused survival strategies that are triggered when schemas related to trauma and unmet needs are activated. These include flight (avoidance), fight (overcompensation), and freeze (surrender).
  - Avoidant protector
  - Overcompensator
  - Compliant surrenderer

- **Innate child modes:** Schema-triggered reactions in adulthood related to childhood unmet needs
  - Vulnerable child
  - Impulsive or undisciplined child
  - Angry child

Unmet Core Childhood Needs and Their Associated Schema Modes

- Lack of secure attachment

  - **Vulnerable child:** The experience of intense loneliness, fear anxiety, sadness

- Lack of validation of feelings and needs, guidance, self-control, and realistic limits

  - **Angry child:** Anger due to perceived unfair treatment or unmet needs

  - **Impulsive/undisciplined child:** Reactively acts on personal desires, with no regard to other's needs or limits

- Rejection and suppression of any core need, in particular love, validation, praise, acceptance, and guidance

  - **Punitive critic:** Harshly punishes and rejects self

  - **Demanding critic:** Pressures self to achieve unreasonably high expectations

- Any unmet childhood need can produce Maladaptive Coping Modes

  - **Avoidant protector:** Breaks relational connections, isolates, physically avoids, withdraws, dissociates

  - **Overcompensator:** Does the opposite of the early maladaptive schema as a coping style to counterattack and control; may be somewhat adaptive at times (e.g., perfectionistic overcontroller at work)

  - **Compliant surrender:** Acts as if the schema is true, surrendering to it. For example, in the defectiveness/shame schema, gives up and accepts self as without worth

- Any unmet childhood need can lead to an underdeveloped healthy adult mode

  - **Healthy adult (underdeveloped):** Meets one's needs in a healthy and mature manner, enjoying pleasures, maintaining healthy bonds, and fulfilling adult life requirements

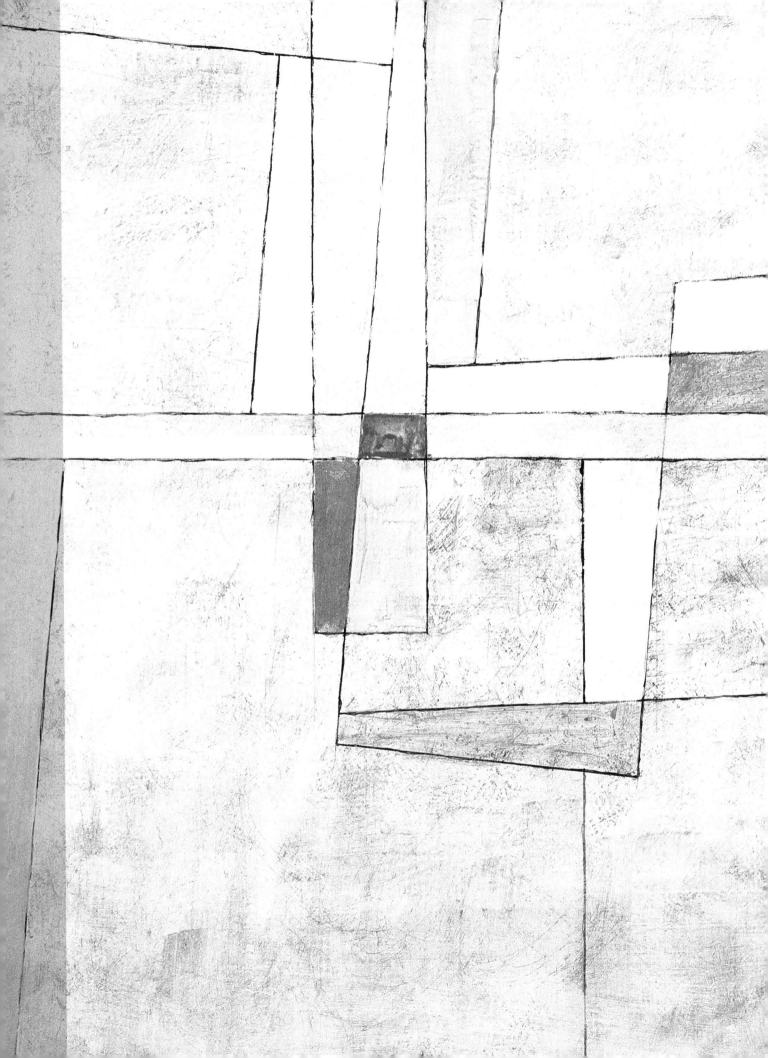

Sample Schema Therapy Syllabus With Embedded Deliberate Practice Exercises

This appendix provides a sample one-semester, three-unit course dedicated to teaching schema therapy (ST). This course is appropriate for graduate students (master's and doctoral) at all levels of training, including first-year students who have not yet worked with clients. We present it as a model that can be adapted to a specific program's contexts and needs. For example, instructors may borrow portions of it to use in other courses, in practica, in didactic training events at externships and internships, in workshops, and in continuing education for postgraduate therapists.

Course Title: Schema Therapy: Theory and Deliberate Practice

Course Description

This course teaches the theory, principles, and core skills of ST. As a course with both didactic and practicum elements, it will review the theoretical model of ST and its change process, the therapist style and intervention of limited reparenting, and the treatment outcome research supporting the effectiveness of the ST approach, and it will foster the use of deliberate practice to enable students to acquire key ST skills.

Course Objectives

Students who complete this course will be able to do the following:

1. Describe the core theory, concepts, and skills of ST
2. Apply the principles of deliberate practice for career-long clinical skill development
3. Demonstrate 12 key ST skills
4. Explain clients' current problems in schema therapy terms
5. Develop client homework corresponding to each session

Date	Lecture and Discussion	Skills Lab	Homework[a]
Week 1	Introduction to schema therapy (ST): theory, history, and research; process and outcome research	Lecture on principles of deliberate practice; deliberate practice research	**To read before Week 1:** Behary et al. (2023, Chapter 1); Young et al. (2003, Chapter 1, pp. 1–62) **Optional reading before Week 1:** Edwards & Arntz (2012, Chapter 1, pp. 3–26); Farrell & Shaw (2022) **Week 1 homework (for next class):** Young et al. (2003, Chapter 6, pp. 177–220); Roediger et al. (2018, Chapter 5, pp. 83–107)
Week 2	Developing a working alliance; bonding and emotional regulation	Exercise 1: Understanding and Attunement	Roediger et al. (2018, Chapter 7, pp. 125–142); Farrell & Shaw (2018, Modules 12 & 20)
Week 3	The healthy adult mode; focus on accessing and supporting client's strengths and abilities	Exercise 2: Supporting and Strengthening the Healthy Adult Mode	Young et al. (2003, Chapters 2 & 3, pp. 63–99)
Week 4	Introducing early maladaptive schemas and their role in current problems	Exercise 3: Schema Education: Beginning to Understand Current Problems in Schema Therapy Terms	Young et al. (2003, Chapter 7, pp. 207–270); Farrell & Shaw (2018, Module 6)
Week 5	Basic concepts of the ST model's etiology of psychological problems	Exercise 4: Linking Unmet Needs, Schema, and Presenting Problem	Young et al. (2018, Chapter 8, pp. 271–305); Roediger et al. (2018, Chapter 4, pp. 57–82)
Week 6	Identifying the role of demanding/punitive inner critic modes in current problems	Exercise 5: Education About Maladaptive Schema Modes	Farrell et al. (2014, pp. 95–98, 267–280); Farrell & Shaw (2018, Module 8)
Week 7	Mode awareness for the maladaptive coping modes	Exercise 6: Recognizing the Mode Shifts of the Maladaptive Coping Modes	Farrell et al. (2014, pp. 99–102); Farrell & Shaw (2018, Module 10)
Week 8	Mode awareness for the demanding/punitive inner critic mode	Exercise 7: Identifying the Presence of the Demanding/Punitive Inner Critic Mode	Farrell et al. (2014, pp. 103–110); Young et al. (2003, Chapters 1 & 2, pp. 4–76); Farrell & Shaw (2018, Module 5)
Week 9	First case conceptualization due (Problem Analysis Plan and Mode Map), self-evaluation, self-reflection	Exercise 14: Mock Schema Therapy Sessions	Farrell et al. (2014, pp. 292–316); Farrell & Shaw (2018, Modules 14 & 15)
Week 10	Mode awareness for the angry and vulnerable child modes	Exercise 8: Identifying the Presence of the Angry and Vulnerable Child Modes	Farrell et al. (2014, pp. 10–15); Roediger et al. (2018, pp. 119–122)
Week 11	Limited reparenting, corrective emotional experiences for the child modes	Exercise 9: Limited Reparenting for the Angry and Vulnerable Child Modes	Farrell et al. (2014, pp. 280–291); Farrell & Shaw (2018, Module 11); Behary (2021, Chapters 7 & 9); Behary (2020, pp. 227–237)
Week 12	Limited reparenting to challenge the demanding/punitive inner critic mode	Exercise 10: Limited Reparenting for the Demanding/Punitive Inner Critic Mode	Roediger et al. (2018, pp. 112–119); Farrell et al. (2014, pp. 267–280); Behary & Dieckmann (2013, Chapter 17)
Week 13	Empathic confrontation	Exercise 11: Limited Reparenting for the Maladaptive Coping Modes: Empathic Confrontation	Young et al. (2003, Chapter 5, pp. 146–176); Farrell & Shaw (2018, Module 11)
Week 14	Mode management and behavioral pattern breaking	Exercise 12: Implementing Behavioral Pattern Breaking Through Homework Assignments	ISST example of case conceptualization
Week 15	Second case conceptualization due, final exam, self-evaluation, skill coaching feedback, self-reflection	Exercise 13: Annotated Schema Therapy Practice Session Transcript	None

Note. ISST = International Society of Schema Therapy.
[a]Homework is for the next class. The citations included are located in the Required Readings section.

Format of Class

Classes are 3 hours long. Course time is split evenly between learning ST theory and acquiring ST skills:

Lecture/Discussion Class: Each week, there will be one Lecture/Discussion class for 1.5 hours focusing on ST theory and related research.

ST Skills Lab: Each week there will be one ST Skills Lab for 1.5 hours. Skills Labs are for practicing ST skills using the exercises in this book. The exercises use therapy simulations (role-plays) with the following goals:

1. Build trainees' skill and confidence for using ST skills with real clients
2. Provide a safe space for experimenting with different therapeutic interventions, without fear of making mistakes
3. Provide plenty of opportunity to explore and "try on" different styles of therapy, so trainees can ultimately discover their own personal, unique therapy style

Mock Sessions: Once in the semester (Week 9), trainees will do a psychotherapy mock session in the ST Skills Lab. In contrast to highly structured and repetitive deliberate practice exercises, a psychotherapy mock session is an unstructured and improvised role-played therapy session. Mock sessions let trainees

1. practice using ST skills responsively,
2. experiment with clinical decision making in an unscripted context,
3. discover their personal therapeutic style, and
4. build endurance for working with real clients.

Homework

Homework will be assigned each week and will include reading, 1 hour of skills practice with an assigned practice partner, and occasional writing assignments. For the skills practice homework, trainees will repeat the exercise they did for that week's ST Skills Lab. Because the instructor will not be there to evaluate performance, trainees should instead complete the Deliberate Practice Reaction Form, as well as the Deliberate Practice Diary Form, for themselves as a self-evaluation.

Case Conceptualization Assignments

Students are to complete two case conceptualizations: one due at midterm and one due at the last day of class. These should be based on the trainees' therapy cases with real clients.

Vulnerability, Privacy, and Boundaries

This course is aimed at developing ST skills, self-awareness, and interpersonal skills in an experiential framework as relevant to clinical work. This course is not psychotherapy or a substitute for psychotherapy. Students should interact at a level of self-disclosure that is personally comfortable and helpful to their own learning. Although becoming aware of internal emotional and psychological processes is necessary for a therapist's development, it is not necessary to reveal all that information to the trainer. It is important for students to sense their own level of safety and privacy. Students are not evaluated on the level of material that they choose to reveal in the class.

In accordance with the *Ethical Principles of Psychologists and Code of Conduct* (American Psychological Association, 2017), students are **not required to disclose personal**

information. Because this class is about developing both interpersonal and ST competence, following are some important points so that students are fully informed as they
make choices to self-disclose:

- Students choose how much, when, and what to disclose. Students are not penalized
  for the choice not to share personal information.

- The learning environment is susceptible to group dynamics much like any other
  group space, and therefore students may be asked to share their observations and
  experiences of the class environment with the singular goal of fostering a more
  inclusive and productive learning environment.

Confidentiality

To create a safe learning environment that is respectful of client and therapist information and diversity and to foster open and vulnerable conversation in class, students are
required to agree to strict confidentiality within and outside of the instruction setting.

Evaluation

Self-Evaluation: At the end of the semester (Week 15), trainees will perform a self-
evaluation. This will help trainees track their progress and identify areas for further
development.

Grading Criteria

As designed, students would be accountable for the level and quality of their performance in

- the Discussion classes,
- the Skills Lab (exercises and mock sessions),
- homework, and
- midterm and final case conceptualizations.

Required Readings

Behary, W. T. (2020). The art of empathic confrontation and limit-setting. In G. Heath &
   H. Startup (Eds.), *Creative methods in schema therapy: Advances and innovation in clinical
   practice* (pp. 227–236). Routledge.

Behary, W. (2021). *Disarming the narcissist* (3rd ed.). New Harbinger Publications.

Behary, W. T., & Dieckmann, E. (2013). Schema therapy for pathological narcissism: The art of
   adaptive reparenting. In J. S. Ogrodniczuk (Ed.), *Understanding and treating pathological
   narcissism* (pp. 285–300). American Psychological Association.

Behary, W. T., Farrell, J. M., Vaz, A., & Rousmaniere, T. (2023). *Deliberate practice in schema
   therapy.* American Psychological Association. https://doi.org/10.1037/0000326-000

Farrell, J. M., Reiss, N., & Shaw, I. A. (2014). *The schema therapy clinician's guide: A complete
   resource for building and delivering individual, group and integrated schema mode
   treatment programs.* John Wiley & Sons. https://doi.org/10.1002/9781118510018

Farrell, J. M., & Shaw, I. A. (2018). *Experiencing schema therapy from the inside out: A self-
   practice/self-reflection workbook for therapists.* Guilford Press.

Roediger, E., Stevens, B. A., & Brockman, R. (2018). *Contextual schema therapy.* New Harbinger
   Publications.

Young, J. E., Klosko, J. S. & Weishaar, M. E. (2003). *Schema therapy: A practitioner's guide.*
   Guilford Press.

Suggested Readings

Behary, W. (2012). Schema therapy for narcissism: A case study. In M. van Vreeswijk, J. Broersen, & M. Nadort (Eds.), *The Wiley-Blackwell handbook of schema therapy: Theory, research, and practice* (pp. 81–90). Wiley-Blackwell.

Behary, W., & Dieckmann, E. (2011). Schema therapy for narcissism: The art of empathic confrontation, limit-setting, and leverage. In W. K. Campbell & J. D. Miller (Eds.), *The handbook of narcissism and narcissistic personality disorder: Theoretical approaches, empirical findings, and treatments* (pp. 445–456). John Wiley & Sons.

Edwards, D., & Arntz, A. (2012). Schema therapy in historical perspective. In M. van Vreeswijk, J. Broersen, & M. Nadort (Eds.), *The Wiley-Blackwell handbook of schema therapy: Theory, research, and practice* (pp. 3–26). Wiley-Blackwell. https://doi.org/10.1002/9781119962830.ch1

Farrell, J., & Shaw, I. A. (2022). Schema therapy: Conceptualization and treatment of personality disorders. In S. K. Huprich (Ed.), *Personality disorders and pathology: Integrating clinical assessment and practice in the DSM-5 and ICD-11 era* (pp. 281–304). American Psychological Association. https://doi.org/10.1037/0000310-013

Rafaeli, E., Bernstein, D. P., & Young, J. (2010). *Schema therapy: Distinctive features.* Routledge. https://doi.org/10.4324/9780203841709

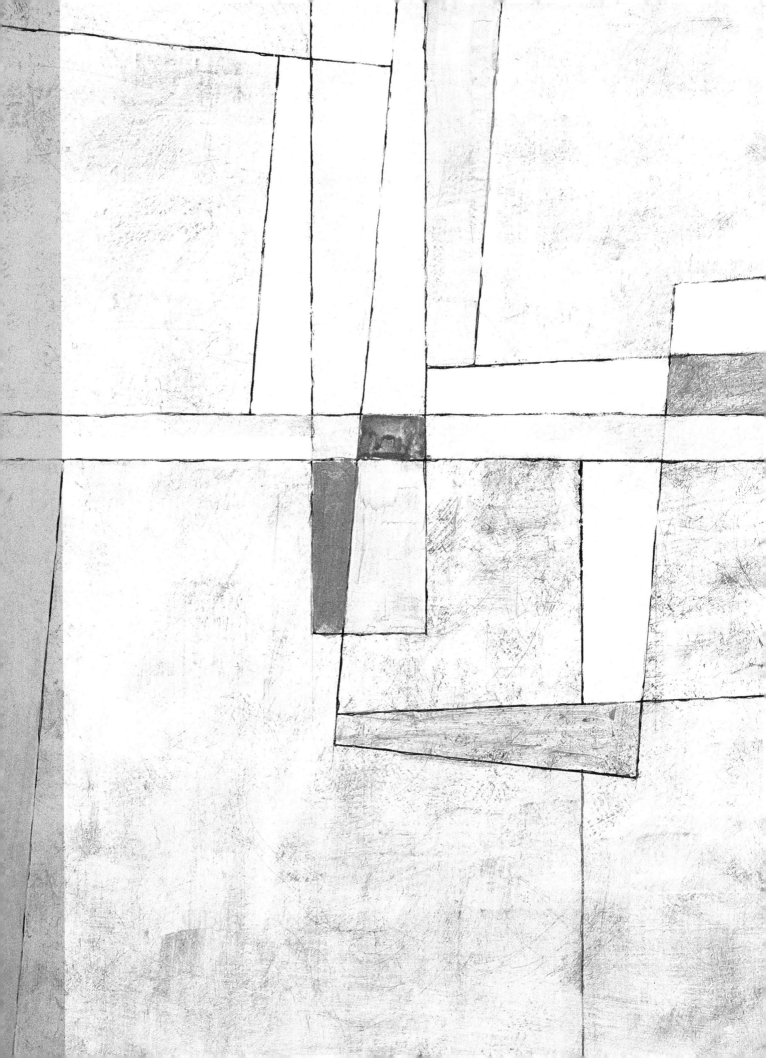

References

American Psychological Association. (2017). *Ethical principles of psychologists and code of conduct* (2002, Amended June 1, 2010, and January 1, 2017). https://www.apa.org/ethics/code/index.aspx

Anderson, T., Ogles, B. M., Patterson, C. L., Lambert, M. J., & Vermeersch, D. A. (2009). Therapist effects: Facilitative interpersonal skills as a predictor of therapist success. *Journal of Clinical Psychology*, *65*(7), 755–768. https://doi.org/10.1002/jclp.20583

Arntz, A. (1994). Borderline personality disorder. In A. T. Beck, A. Freeman, & D. D. Davis (Eds.), *Cognitive therapy for personality disorders* (pp. 187–215). Guilford Press.

Bailey, R. J., & Ogles, B. M. (2019, August 1). Common factors as a therapeutic approach: What is required? *Practice Innovations*, *4*(4), 241–254. https://doi.org/10.1037/pri0000100

Bamelis, L. L., Evers, S. M., Spinhoven, P., & Arntz, A. (2014). Results of a multicenter randomized controlled trial of the clinical effectiveness of schema therapy for personality disorders. *The American Journal of Psychiatry*, *171*(3), 305–322. https://doi.org/10.1176/appi.ajp.2013.12040518

Barlow, D. H. (2010). Negative effects from psychological treatments: A perspective. *American Psychologist*, *65*(1), 13–20. https://doi.org/10.1037/a0015643

Behary, W. T. (2008). *Disarming the narcissist: Surviving and thriving with the self-absorbed.* New Harbinger Publications.

Behary, W. T. (2020). The art of empathic confrontation and limit-setting. In G. Heath & H. Startup (Eds.), *Creative methods in schema therapy: Advances and innovation in clinical practice.* Routledge.

Behary, W. T. (2021). *Disarming the narcissist: Surviving and thriving with the self-absorbed* (3rd ed.). New Harbinger Publications.

Behary, W. T., & Dieckmann, E. (2013). Schema therapy for pathological narcissism: The art of adaptive reparenting. In J. S. Ogrodniczuk (Ed.), *Understanding and treating pathological narcissism* (pp. 285–300). American Psychological Association.

Behary, W. T., Farrell, J. M., Vaz, A., & Rousmaniere, T. (2023). *Deliberate practice in schema therapy.* American Psychological Association. https://doi.org/10.1037/0000326-000

Bennett-Levy, J. (2019). Why therapists should walk the talk: The theoretical and empirical case for personal practice in therapist training and professional development. *Journal of Behavior Therapy and Experimental Psychiatry*, *62*, 133–145. https://doi.org/10.1016/j.jbtep.2018.08.004

Bennett-Levy, J., & Finlay-Jones, A. (2018). The role of personal practice in therapist skill development: A model to guide therapists, educators, supervisors and researchers. *Cognitive Behaviour Therapy*, *47*(3), 185–205. https://doi.org/10.1080/16506073.2018.1434678

Bohart, A. C., & Wade, A. G. (2013). The client in psychotherapy. In M. J. Lambert (Ed.), *Bergin and Garfield's handbook of psychotherapy and behavior change* (6th ed., pp. 219–257). John Wiley & Sons.

Bugatti, M., & Boswell, J. F. (2016). Clinical errors as a lack of context responsiveness. *Psychotherapy: Theory, Research, & Practice, 53*(3), 262–267. https://doi.org/10.1037/pst0000080

Cassidy, J., & Shaver, P. R. (Eds.). (1999). *Handbook of attachment: Theory, research, and clinical applications* (pp. 21–43). Guilford Press.

Castonguay, L. G., Goldfried, M. R., Wiser, S., Raue, P. J., & Hayes, A. M. (1996). Predicting the effect of cognitive therapy for depression: A study of unique and common factors. *Journal of Consulting and Clinical Psychology, 64*(3), 497–504. https://doi.org/10.1037/0022-006X.64.3.497

Coker, J. (1990). *How to practice jazz.* Jamey Aebersold.

Cook, R. (2005). *It's about that time: Miles Davis on and off record.* Atlantic Books.

Csikszentmihalyi, M. (1997). *Finding flow: The psychology of engagement with everyday life.* HarperCollins.

de Klerk, N., Abma, T. A., Bamelis, L. L., & Arntz, A. (2017). Schema therapy for personality disorders: A qualitative study of patients' and therapists' perspectives. *Behavioural and Cognitive Psychotherapy, 45*(1), 31–45. https://doi.org/10.1017/S1352465816000357

Edwards, D., & Arntz, A. (2012). Schema therapy in historical perspective. In M. van Vreeswijk, J. Broersen, & M. Nadort (Eds.), *The Wiley-Blackwell handbook of schema therapy: Theory, research, and practice* (pp. 3–26). Wiley-Blackwell. https://doi.org/10.1002/9781119962830.ch1

Ellis, M. V., Berger, L., Hanus, A. E., Ayala, E. E., Swords, B. A., & Siembor, M. (2014). Inadequate and harmful clinical supervision: Testing a revised framework and assessing occurrence. *The Counseling Psychologist, 42*(4), 434–472. https://doi.org/10.1177/0011000013508656

Ericsson, K. A. (2003). Development of elite performance and deliberate practice: An update from the perspective of the expert performance approach. In J. L. Starkes & K. A. Ericsson (Eds.), *Expert performance in sports: Advances in research on sport expertise* (pp. 49–83). Human Kinetics.

Ericsson, K. A. (2004). Deliberate practice and the acquisition and maintenance in medicine and related domains: Invited address. *Academic Medicine, 79*, S70–S81. https://doi.org/10.1097/00001888-200410001-00022

Ericsson, K. A. (2006). The influence of experience and deliberate practice on the development of superior expert performance. In K. A. Ericsson, N. Charness, P. J. Feltovich, & R. R. Hoffman (Eds.), *The Cambridge handbook of expertise and expert performance* (pp. 683–703). Cambridge University Press. https://doi.org/10.1017/CBO9780511816796.038

Ericsson, K. A., Hoffman, R. R., Kozbelt, A., & Williams, A. M. (Eds.). (2018). *The Cambridge handbook of expertise and expert performance* (2nd ed.). Cambridge University Press. https://doi.org/10.1017/9781316480748

Ericsson, K. A., Krampe, R. T., & Tesch-Römer, C. (1993). The role of deliberate practice in the acquisition of expert performance. *Psychological Review, 100*(3), 363–406. https://doi.org/10.1037/0033-295X.100.3.363

Ericsson, K. A., & Pool, R. (2016). *Peak: Secrets from the new science of expertise.* Houghton Mifflin Harcourt.

Farrell, J. M., Reiss, N., & Shaw, I. A. (2014). *The schema therapy clinician's guide: A complete resource for building and delivering individual, group and integrated schema mode treatment programs.* John Wiley & Sons. https://doi.org/10.1002/9781118510018

Farrell, J. M., & Shaw, I. A. (1994). Emotional awareness training: A prerequisite to effective cognitive-behavioral treatment of borderline personality disorder. *Cognitive and Behavioral Practice, 1*(1), 71–91. https://doi.org/10.1016/S1077-7229(05)80087-2

Farrell, J. M., & Shaw, I. A. (Eds.). (2012). *Group schema therapy for borderline personality disorder: A step-by-step treatment manual with patient workbook.* Wiley-Blackwell. https://doi.org/10.1002/9781119943167

Farrell, J. M., & Shaw, I. A. (2018). *Experiencing schema therapy from the inside out: A self-practice/self-reflection workbook for therapists.* Guilford Press.

Farrell, J., & Shaw, I. A. (2022). Schema therapy: Conceptualization and treatment of personality disorders. In S. K. Huprich (Ed.), *Personality disorders and pathology: Integrating clinical assessment and practice in the* DSM-5 *and* ICD-11 *era* (pp. 281–304). American Psychological Association. https://doi.org/10.1037/0000310-013

Farrell, J. M., Shaw, I. A., & Webber, M. A. (2009). A schema-focused approach to group psychotherapy for outpatients with borderline personality disorder: A randomized controlled trial. *Journal of Behavior Therapy and Experimental Psychiatry*, 40(2), 317–328. https://doi.org/10.1016/j.jbtep.2009.01.002

Fisher, R. P., & Craik, F. I. M. (1977). Interaction between encoding and retrieval operations in cued recall. *Journal of Experimental Psychology: Human Learning and Memory*, 3(6), 701–711. https://doi.org/10.1037/0278-7393.3.6.701

Giesen-Bloo, J., van Dyck, R., Spinhoven, P., van Tilburg, W., Dirksen, C., van Asselt, T., Kremers, I., Nadort, M., Arntz, A., Nadort, M., & Arntz, A. (2006). Outpatient psychotherapy for borderline personality disorder: Randomized trial of schema-focused therapy vs transference-focused psychotherapy. *Archives of General Psychiatry*, 63(6), 649–658. https://doi.org/10.1001/archpsyc.63.6.649

Gladwell, M. (2008). *Outliers: The story of success*. Little, Brown & Company.

Goldberg, S. B., Babins-Wagner, R., Rousmaniere, T., Berzins, S., Hoyt, W. T., Whipple, J. L., Miller, S. D., & Wampold, B. E. (2016). Creating a climate for therapist improvement: A case study of an agency focused on outcomes and deliberate practice. *Psychotherapy: Theory, Research, & Practice*, 53(3), 367–375. https://doi.org/10.1037/pst0000060

Goldberg, S., Rousmaniere, T. G., Miller, S. D., Whipple, J., Nielsen, S. L., Hoyt, W., & Wampold, B. E. (2016). Do psychotherapists improve with time and experience? A longitudinal analysis of outcomes in a clinical setting. *Journal of Counseling Psychology*, 63, 1–11. https://doi.org/10.1037/cou0000131

Goldman, R. N., Vaz, A., & Rousmaniere, T. (2021). *Deliberate practice in emotion-focused therapy*. American Psychological Association. https://doi.org/10.1037/0000227-000

Goodyear, R. K. (2015). Using accountability mechanisms more intentionally: A framework and its implications for training professional psychologists. *American Psychologist*, 70(8), 736–743. https://doi.org/10.1037/a0039828

Goodyear, R. K., & Nelson, M. L. (1997). The major formats of psychotherapy supervision. In C. E. Watkins, Jr. (Ed.), *Handbook of psychotherapy supervision*. Wiley.

Goodyear, R. K., & Rousmaniere, T. G. (2017). Helping therapists to each day become a little better than they were the day before: The expertise-development model of supervision and consultation. In T. G. Rousmaniere, R. Goodyear, S. D. Miller, & B. Wampold (Eds.), *The cycle of excellence: Using deliberate practice to improve supervision and training* (pp. 67–95). John Wiley & Sons. https://doi.org/10.1002/9781119165590.ch4

Goodyear, R. K., Wampold, B. E., Tracey, T. J., & Lichtenberg, J. W. (2017). Psychotherapy expertise should mean superior outcomes and demonstrable improvement over time. *The Counseling Psychologist*, 45(1), 54–65. https://doi.org/10.1177/0011000016652691

Haggerty, G., & Hilsenroth, M. J. (2011). The use of video in psychotherapy supervision. *British Journal of Psychotherapy*, 27(2), 193–210. https://doi.org/10.1111/j.1752-0118.2011.01232.x

Hatcher, R. L. (2015). Interpersonal competencies: Responsiveness, technique, and training in psychotherapy. *American Psychologist*, 70(8), 747–757. https://doi.org/10.1037/a0039803

Henry, W. P., Strupp, H. H., Butler, S. F., Schacht, T. E., & Binder, J. L. (1993). Effects of training in time-limited dynamic psychotherapy: Changes in therapist behavior. *Journal of Consulting and Clinical Psychology*, 61(3), 434–440. https://doi.org/10.1037/0022-006X.61.3.434

Hill, C. E., Kivlighan, D. M., III, Rousmaniere, T., Kivlighan, D. M., Jr., Gerstenblith, J., & Hillman, J. (2020). Deliberate practice for the skill of immediacy: A multiple case study of doctoral student therapists and clients. *Psychotherapy: Theory, Research, & Practice*, 57(4), 587–597. https://doi.org/10.1037/pst0000247

Hill, C. E., & Knox, S. (2013). Training and supervision in psychotherapy: Evidence for effective practice. In M. J. Lambert (Ed.), *Handbook of psychotherapy and behavior change* (6th ed., pp. 775–811). John Wiley & Sons.

Kendall, P. C., & Beidas, R. S. (2007). Smoothing the trail for dissemination of evidence-based practices for youth: Flexibility within fidelity. *Professional Psychology, Research and Practice*, 38(1), 13–19. https://doi.org/10.1037/0735-7028.38.1.13

Kendall, P. C., & Frank, H. E. (2018). Implementing evidence-based treatment protocols: Flexibility within fidelity. *Clinical Psychology: Science and Practice, 25*(4), e12271. https://doi.org/10.1111/cpsp.12271

Koziol, L. F., & Budding, D. E. (2012). Procedural learning. In N. M. Seel (Ed.), *Encyclopedia of the sciences of learning* (pp. 2694–2696). Springer. https://doi.org/10.1007/978-1-4419-1428-6_670

Lambert, M. J. (2010). Yes, it is time for clinicians to monitor treatment outcome. In B. L. Duncan, S. C. Miller, B. E. Wampold, & M. A. Hubble (Eds.), *Heart and soul of change: Delivering what works in therapy* (2nd ed., pp. 239–266). American Psychological Association. https://doi.org/10.1037/12075-008

Markman, K. D., & Tetlock, P. E. (2000). Accountability and close-call counterfactuals: The loser who nearly won and the winner who nearly lost. *Personality and Social Psychology Bulletin, 26*(10), 1213–1224. https://doi.org/10.1177/0146167200262004

McGaghie, W. C., Issenberg, S. B., Barsuk, J. H., & Wayne, D. B. (2014). A critical review of simulation-based mastery learning with translational outcomes. *Medical Education, 48*(4), 375–385. https://doi.org/10.1111/medu.12391

McLeod, J. (2017). Qualitative methods for routine outcome measurement. In T. G. Rousmaniere, R. Goodyear, D. D. Miller, & B. E. Wampold (Eds.), *The cycle of excellence: Using deliberate practice to improve supervision and training* (pp. 99–122). John Wiley & Sons. https://doi.org/10.1002/9781119165590.ch5

Norcross, J. C., & Guy, J. D. (2005). The prevalence and parameters of personal therapy in the United States. In J. D. Geller, J. C. Norcross, & D. E. Orlinsky (Eds.), *The psychotherapist's own psychotherapy: Patient and clinician perspectives* (pp. 165–176). Oxford University Press.

Norcross, J. C., Lambert, M. J., & Wampold, B. E. (2019). *Psychotherapy relationships that work* (3rd ed.). Oxford University Press.

Orlinsky, D. E., & Ronnestad, M. H. (2005). *How psychotherapists develop.* American Psychological Association.

Owen, J., & Hilsenroth, M. J. (2014). Treatment adherence: The importance of therapist flexibility in relation to therapy outcomes. *Journal of Counseling Psychology, 61*(2), 280–288. https://doi.org/10.1037/a0035753

Prescott, D. S., Maeschalck, C. L., & Miller, S. D. (Eds.). (2017). *Feedback-informed treatment in clinical practice: Reaching for excellence.* American Psychological Association. https://doi.org/10.1037/0000039-000

Rafaeli, E., Bernstein, D. P., & Young, J. (2010). *Schema therapy: Distinctive features.* Routledge. https://doi.org/10.4324/9780203841709

Roediger, E., Stevens, B. A., & Brockman, R. (2018). *Contextual schema therapy.* New Harbinger Publications.

Rousmaniere, T. G. (2016). Deliberate practice for psychotherapists: A guide to improving clinical effectiveness. Routledge Press/Taylor & Francis. https://doi.org/10.4324/9781315472256

Rousmaniere, T. G. (2019). *Mastering the inner skills of psychotherapy: A deliberate practice handbook.* Gold Lantern Press.

Rousmaniere, T. G., Goodyear, R., Miller, S. D., & Wampold, B. E. (Eds.). (2017). *The cycle of excellence: Using deliberate practice to improve supervision and training.* John Wiley & Sons. https://doi.org/10.1002/9781119165590

Siegel, D. J. (1999). *The developing mind.* Guilford Press.

Smith, S. M. (1979). Remembering in and out of context. *Journal of Experimental Psychology: Human Learning and Memory, 5*(5), 460–471. https://doi.org/10.1037/0278-7393.5.5.460

Squire, L. R. (2004). Memory systems of the brain: A brief history and current perspective. *Neurobiology of Learning and Memory, 82*(3), 171–177. https://doi.org/10.1016/j.nlm.2004.06.005

Stiles, W. B., Honos-Webb, L., & Surko, M. (1998). Responsiveness in psychotherapy. *Clinical Psychology: Science and Practice, 5*(4), 439–458. https://doi.org/10.1111/j.1468-2850.1998.tb00166.x

Stiles, W. B., & Horvath, A. O. (2017). Appropriate responsiveness as a contribution to therapist effects. In L. G. Castonguay & C. E. Hill (Eds.), *How and why are some therapists better than others? Understanding therapist effects* (pp. 71–84). American Psychological Association. https://doi.org/10.1037/0000034-005

Taylor, J. M., & Neimeyer, G. J. (2017). Lifelong professional improvement: The evolution of continuing education: Past, present, and future. In T. G. Rousmaniere, R. Goodyear, S. D. Miller, & B. Wampold (Eds.), *The cycle of excellence: Using deliberate practice to improve supervision and training* (pp. 219–248). John Wiley & Sons.

Tracey, T. J. G., Wampold, B. E., Goodyear, R. K., & Lichtenberg, J. W. (2015). Improving expertise in psychotherapy. *Psychotherapy Bulletin, 50*(1), 7–13.

Wass, R., & Golding, C. (2014). Sharpening a tool for teaching: The zone of proximal development. *Teaching in Higher Education, 19*(6), 671–684. https://doi.org/10.1080/13562517.2014.901958

Younan, R., Farrell, J., & May, T. (2018). "Teaching me to parent myself": The feasibility of an in-patient group schema therapy programme for complex trauma. *Behavioural and Cognitive Psychotherapy, 46*(4), 463–478. https://doi.org/10.1017/S1352465817000698

Young, J. E. (1990). *Cognitive therapy for personality disorder: A schema focused approach.* Professional Resource Exchange.

Young, J. E., Klosko, J. S., & Weishaar, M. E. (2003). *Schema therapy: A practitioner's guide.* Guilford Press.

Zaretskii, V. (2009). The zone of proximal development: What Vygotsky did not have time to write. *Journal of Russian & East European Psychology, 47*(6), 70–93. https://doi.org/10.2753/RPO1061-0405470604

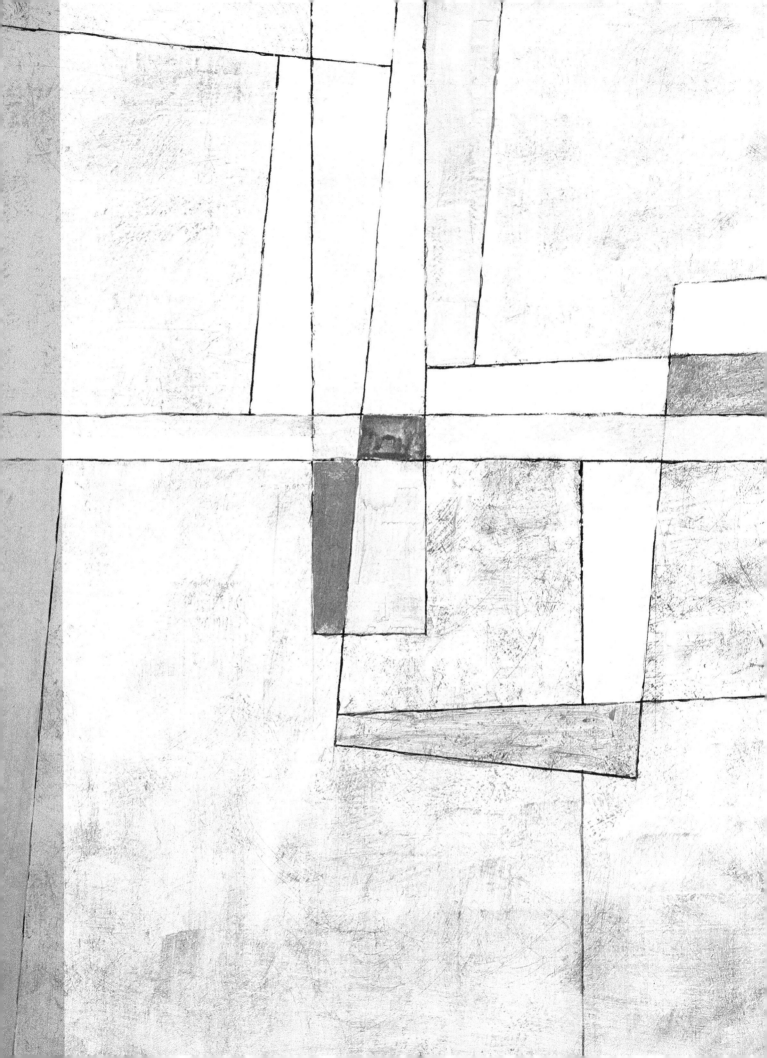

Index

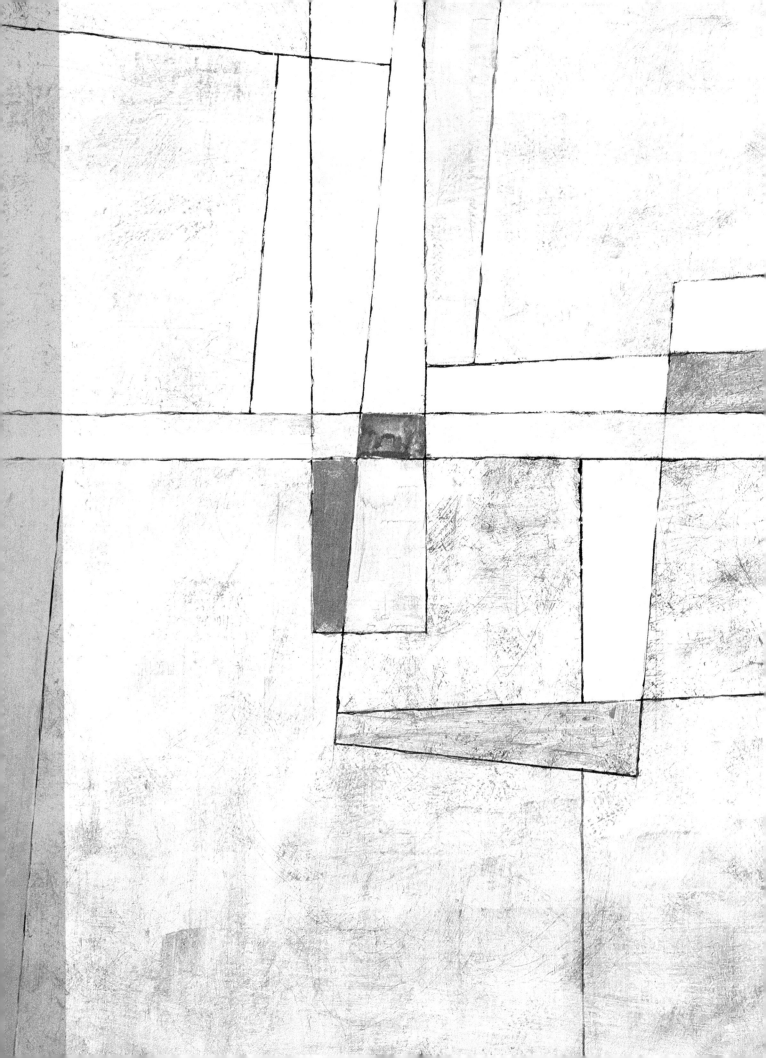

About the Authors

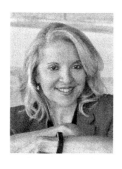

Wendy T. Behary, MSW, LCSW, is the founder and director of The Cognitive Therapy Center of New Jersey and The Schema Therapy Institutes of NJ-NYC-DC. She was also the president of the International Society of Schema Therapy from 2010 to 2014. She is the author of *Disarming the Narcissist: Surviving and Thriving With the Self-Absorbed* (New Harbinger Publications), now translated into 15 languages. She has been treating narcissist clients, partners, and other people dealing with them, and couples experiencing relationship problems; training professionals; and supervising psychotherapists for more than 20 years. She lectures both nationally and internationally to professional and general audiences on the subjects of schema therapy and of narcissism and relationships.

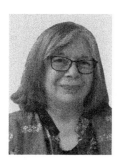

Joan M. Farrell, PhD, is a licensed clinical psychologist and the research director of the Center for Borderline Personality Disorder Treatment and Research, Indiana University–Purdue University Indianapolis (IUPUI). She is an adjunct professor of psychology at IUPUI and was on the clinical psychology faculty in the Department of Psychiatry at Indiana University School of Medicine for 25 years. Dr. Farrell was the coordinator for training and certification on the executive board of the International Society of Schema Therapy (2012–2018). She is the developer, with Ida Shaw, of a group model of schema therapy, which integrates experiential interventions and harnesses the therapeutic factors of groups. Together they also wrote two books on this model for borderline and other personality disorders. Their latest book is *Experiencing Schema Therapy From the Inside Out: A Self-Practice/Self-Reflection Workbook for Therapists* (Guilford Press). Dr. Farrell provides schema therapy training and self-practice/self-reflection workshops nationally and internationally.

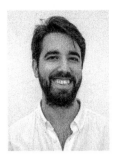

Alexandre Vaz, PhD, is cofounder and chief academic officer of Sentio University, Los Angeles, California. He provides deliberate practice workshops and advanced clinical training and supervision to clinicians around the world. Dr. Vaz is the author/coeditor of multiple books on deliberate practice and psychotherapy training and two series of clinical training books: The Essentials of Deliberate Practice (American Psychological Association) and Advanced Therapeutics, Clinical and Interpersonal Skills (Elsevier). He has held multiple committee roles for the Society for the Exploration of Psychotherapy Integration and the Society for Psychotherapy Research. Dr. Vaz is founder and host of "Psychotherapy Expert Talks," an acclaimed interview series with distinguished psychotherapists and therapy researchers.

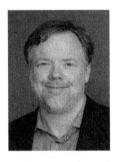

Tony Rousmaniere, PsyD, is cofounder and program director of Sentio University, Los Angeles, California. He provides workshops, webinars, and advanced clinical training and supervision to clinicians around the world. Dr. Rousmaniere is the author/coeditor of multiple books on deliberate practice and psychotherapy training and two series of clinical training books: The Essentials of Deliberate Practice (American Psychological Association) and Advanced Therapeutics, Clinical and Interpersonal Skills (Elsevier). In 2017, he published the widely cited article "What Your Therapist Doesn't Know" in *The Atlantic Monthly*. Dr. Rousmaniere supports the open-data movement and publishes his aggregated clinical outcome data, in deidentified form, on his website (https://drtonyr.com/). A Fellow of the American Psychological Association, Dr. Rousmaniere was awarded the Early Career Award by the Society for the Advancement of Psychotherapy (APA Division 29).